TIME IS COWS
TIMELESS WISDOM
OF THE MAASAI

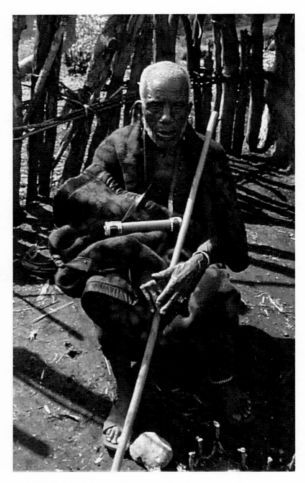

Lekoko Ole Sululu's father at his home in the Ngorongoro Conservation Area, Tanzania

TANYA PERGOLA Ph.D.

TIME IS COWS
TIMELESS WISDOM
OF THE MAASAI

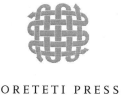

ORETETI PRESS

Tanya Pergola, www.tanyapergola.com

Design by Hans Teensma, www.impressinc.com

Cover photograph by Andreas Sigrist, www.andreassigrist.com

ISBN: 978-0-9911910-1-7

Co-printed in the United States of America and in South Africa

This book is dedicated to my father,
Charles Pergola, who inspired me to love life,
to understand how healing makes our hearts
happy, and, to treasure all the lessons in life
that make us grow and blossom.

And to the Maasai, who entrusted me
to find a way to share their rapidly
disappearing indigenous knowledge
so their enduring wisdom can
help heal a troubled world.
I humbly hope that I have met
your expectations.

Contents

"Don't gain the world and lose your soul. Wisdom is better than silver and gold."

—Bob Marley

I.

Setting the Stage

THE BIRTHPLACE

I have a heart for indigenous people. When I meet someone who has a deep connection to her ancestral past and a direct line into the earth, something sparks between us. We connect on an elemental level. The voice of Mother Nature speaks through us, even while we are dressed in human costumes.

On a bright Sunday more than a decade ago, I found myself in a primordial forest at the bottom of Ngorongoro Crater in Tanzania, accompanied by elephants, eagles, and Maasai warriors who have been at home in that remarkable region for many millennia. As I looked at the high canopy of trees surrounding me, their leaves began to shimmer, to *sparkle,* and an overwhelming sensation came over me. Everything was profoundly *alive.* And I sensed that I had come to a place on planet earth that could teach me wondrous things.

As a social anthropologist, I was aware, of course, that I was only steps away from Oldapai Gorge—ancient terrain where our human ancestors took *their* very first steps. Yet something else about that place drew me in as well, pulling at my intellect as well as my soul. My brain twitched. My heart danced. I was filled with delicious anticipation, and I sensed that whatever I was about to learn would be so unique, so *important*, that I would be compelled to share it with members of my own tribe.

On that singular Sunday, I simply and very powerfully knew that what I would learn there would be a kind of antidote to the stresses, challenges, and many enigmas of our complex contemporary lives. I was about to take an extraordinary journey back to my roots—to the roots of us all. In equatorial Africa, I would re-

On the crater floor, Ngorongoro, Tanzania

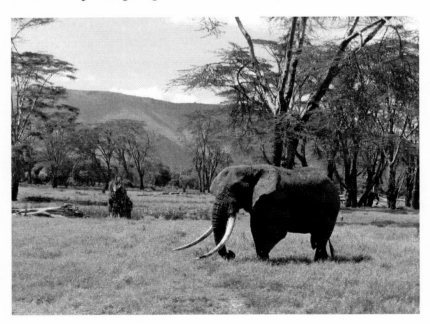

learn what it means to be human, and would discover a wonderful medicine for healing ourselves and our communities using the eternal forces of nature.

What a journey! And what remarkable lessons I learned beginning that day! I'm eager to share them with you.

MY GLOBAL ROOTS

I was born in Connecticut, not far from New York City. My father's family had emigrated from Sicily in the 1920s. My mother was born in what is now Azerbaijan and was raised in northern Italy. So, I was born a global girl, and my bloodlines and the cultural influences inside my childhood home were deliciously mixed, often making for excellent culinary experiences—from the homemade ravioli we would have on special Sundays to the exotic *piroschki* I would take in my lunchbox to school.

Yet when it came to gaining clarity about some of life's biggest questions—Who am I? What do I want?—I was often met with a flood of perplexing answers. The prevailing belief in Fairfield County, Connecticut in the 1980s was that, in order to be successful, a young woman should go to university, do well, and continue paving the way for other women that first was cleared by the women's movement of the 1960s. Having been born with a pioneering spirit, this plan seemed reasonable.

But my father, who as a good Sicilian had originally hoped I would be born a boy, spoke to me as if I *were* his son, and he plainly enjoyed criticizing the feminists he knew and, by extension therefore, me. Deep down, however, I knew that by biological and socio-logical default I was necessarily a "feminist," and the cultural buffet of sometimes conflicting ideas from my earliest days certainly did provide many interesting meals on my life's plate.

A born peacemaker, when disparate ideas come my way I instinctively start building bridges. On a practical level, I think nothing of serving Italian wine with a Russian meal; and on more spiritual and philosophical levels, I have often found myself seeking the common ground between my Muslim, Christian, and Jewish friends. A born optimist, I try to seek out the good in everyone and everything, and create combinations of the best of two or more worlds.

Perhaps inevitably, at university I abandoned the majors my father had chosen for me—marketing and advertising—for anthropology and sociology. In those departments I truly fell in love with reading and learning for the very first time in my life. As I read about the bushmen of the Kalahari, I delighted to im-agine what it would be like to live life in a manner so different from my own. In my social psychology classes I freed my mind to explore the vast realms in which society and culture co-create self and identity. I discovered that we are who we are because of our relationships with those around us. And as each of us acts and reacts to the world we encounter, we make changes—individually and collectively.

I was hooked, and I dove in deeply enough that I eventually earned a Ph.D. in sociology at one of the most exciting places I could have been at the time, the University of Washington in Seattle. 1990s Seattle was the talk of the nation, if not the world.

With its contribution to music—the grunge rock of Nirvana and other great bands—the technology revolution spurred by local behemoth Microsoft and dozens of lesser companies that spun in its orbit, and the coffee craze that was initiated by a hometown roasting company called Starbucks, Seattle and the Pacific Northwest were ground zero for an emerging new world. The city of Seattle launched one of the first extensive recycling programs in the country; Bastyr, one of the first natural medicine universities was located in Puget Sound, and the region was a national leader in "new age" religion. My friends and I liked to think of ourselves as "post-modern" folks, living with our fingers on the pulse of, well, we weren't entirely sure, but we knew at the very least that people around the world were awfully interested in what we were saying and doing.

But with this onslaught of creativity came traffic jams and a quickening of the pace of life that felt a little unnatural. It sometimes felt like my fellow urbanites and I were skating on ice not yet hard enough to support us. I remember one evening in 1998 talking with a university colleague about the very risky decisions of several friends we shared to max out multiple credit cards with no real plan to pay them off, as well as buying houses they clearly could not afford.

The two of us came to the conclusion that the American economy was a kind of "vapor," capable of being clearly seen for what it is from a bit of distance, but which disappears when you're inside of it. We guessed the economy would roll along recklessly for about ten more years, and then it would encounter some monumental challenges. And with all the extraordinary advances in technology, financial growth, and health care, were we not forgetting some basic, even elemental aspects of our humanity? So many people appeared to be running around like headless chickens, and people's physical and mental health seemed to be getting collectively worse rather than better.

Trained as a pharmacist in the 1950s, my father loved trying to help family and friends get well and stay well, and I remember many conversations with him about which medicines really could cure pain and suffering. He told me that he and his classmates at the University of Connecticut had been required to study botany, but that later botany had been dropped from the curriculum, and how delighted he was to learn that botany was being taught again to pharmacy students. Plants, he was certain, held *many* benefits for human health.

There was a small closet in my childhood home that held dozens of samples of pills and potions my father obtained at pharmaceutical conferences and the trade events he attended—although that closet was seldom opened. My sister and I rarely got sick, neither did my parents, and I now understand that a primary reason for our collective good health was my mother's insistence on serving fresh, homemade Italian meals. She was raised with the belief that "food is medicine," and that if you ate well, other treatments were rarely needed. Inspired by my now-deceased father, who understood the efficacious qualities of plants, and by my mother's dedication to creating delicious and healthy food, I realize today that I was nurtured by them and was perfectly poised for the leap into the waters of nature healing that, unbeknownst to me, I was about to undertake.

AFRICA CALLING

I had a phone in my hand and was about to call and cancel my booking with the American travel company that was organizing my journey to Tanzania—the trip that would take me to the summit of Mount Kilimanjaro, on a wildlife safari, and then to the exotic island of Zanzibar. Lately I had become afraid that I just didn't have the energy to get myself half way around the world and up a 19,340 foot mountain.

I was not well—on all levels, physically, emotionally, and spiritually. For almost two years, I gradually had been getting sicker. When my father died in 1997, I had failed to truly grieve his loss in my life. Instead, I followed a rather more common American strategy by filling the void I felt with intensive career-focused work, completing my doctoral thesis while working full-time as a consultant for a start-up firm that was capitalizing on Americans' rising interest in holistic health and wellness.

Imagine the irony: my job was to help companies capitalize on people's growing fascination with eating and living more healthfully, and in the process I was making myself less and less well. Yet even though I was truly exhausted and about to call and cancel my trip, I ultimately hesitated and put down the phone. I don't know why.

A few days later, however, the travel company called me, explaining that a large family group had cancelled its booking, meaning that the journey I was scheduled to be part of would have to be cancelled. But the travel consultant wondered whether I would be interested in joining another group, one scheduled to depart for

Tanzania a few weeks after the original date of my booking.

I considered: this was my chance to get out of the whole thing and not lose a dime in deposits, because the cancellation wasn't my fault. But instead of doing exactly that, I astonished myself by merrily announcing, "Sure! No problem, sign me up for the later departure."

In retrospect, it's clear: something beyond my rational mind led my exhausted self to the airplane that ferried me to East Africa for the first time. Whatever it was, I am blessed that I can now share the story. It's a story that goes far beyond the stark headlines of disease, death, conflict, and poverty in Africa. It's a tale, rather, about life, wellness, co-creation, and riches. I received a second Ph.D. in Tanzania—but this one did not involve reading books or taking classes or writing a dissertation.

Yet it did involve many profound lessons and an array of very difficult tests—trials of the mind as well as of the heart.

PLANTING SEEDS

My African adventure may have begun on the summit of Mt. Kilimanjaro, but the real journey began when I returned to the United States. I arrived back in Seattle in early October 1999, and in more ways than one, I was out of sorts. What a case of poor planning I had done: two days before I'd been sunning on the beach in Zanzibar, and now here I was, waking wrapped up in a down duvet and listening to the rain steadily fall on the roof of my Seattle home.

Dressed in wool and fleece, I headed over to the University of Washington, where I was advising students in the Environmental

Studies program. On the way to an appointment, I stopped at the university bookstore, hoping to find some comfort in old, familiar surroundings. I studied a wall of books written by authors scheduled to speak in Seattle in the coming weeks. Every other title seemed to have something to do with "individual freedom," "self-help," or "becoming independent." My sour mood worsened when I thought, "What's so great about working hard enough to survive completely alone in this world?" Sure, the foundational values of freedom and liberty that are forged into the American psyche are important, but had we gone too far? What were we freeing ourselves from? Was it making us any happier?

Later that day, one of the co-directors of the Environmental Studies program overheard me sharing with a student some of my experiences with wildlife management and traditional communities in Tanzania and he stopped and asked, "Tanya, are you going to listen to Wangari Maathai speak this evening?"

"What? She's here?" I replied. And the day instantly began to improve.

I had been a big fan of Wangari's work with women in Kenya for some time. A number of the books I had read on the environmental movement and ways to curb radical climate change mentioned the organization she founded, The Greenbelt Movement. Wangari had left her position as a professor at the University of Nairobi to work at the grassroots, helping to empower women, psychologically and economically, and had brilliantly focused on planting trees as the primary means to do so. (Twenty-seven years and thirty million trees later, Wangari and the Greenbelt Movement would be awarded the Noble Peace Prize in 2004.)

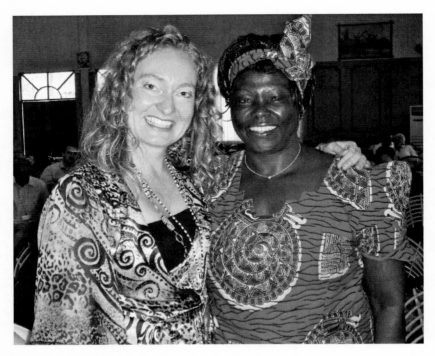

Wangari Maathai and I in Arusha in 2008,
three years before she passed away

But in 1999, what in the world was this wonderful woman doing in Seattle? The University of Washington wasn't known to be
particularly strong in the field of African Studies at the time. But
my colleague explained that Wangari was also participating at a
workshop on African issues on nearby Whidbey Island the following weekend. He was on the board of the organization hosting the
event, he said, and he would be happy to inquire whether I could
attend as well. I'd be delighted, I told him. It would be lovely to
be in the presence of such interesting people—and to connect to
Africa again as the long and rainy Northwest winter commenced.

I hadn't truly had a role model since I was twelve and Nadia
Comaneci, the young Romanian, had been the first gymnast ever to
receive a perfect score of ten in the Olympics—something an aspir-
ing gymnast like me believed was a super-human achievement.

When Wangari Maathai walked into the room at the university that evening, it was as if Mother Earth herself entered.
Her face glowed and her eyes had the intensity and sparkle I
remembered seeing in many of the people I recently had met
in Tanzania. Wangari had been the first East African woman to
receive a Ph.D. Her own bloodline was Kikuyu-Maasai, and she
spoke phrases similar to those I had been using in my Environmental Studies and Social Change courses: "We don't need any
more research. We know what is wrong. We need to act." That
evening, Wangari seemed to cut down all the ongoing debates
on development aid, foreign policy in the Third World, and ways
to heal from colonialism with a scythe and got right to the point.
We simply needed to plant more trees. It had been a very long
time since I had been so inspired.

I walked up to Wangari after her talk and began a conversation. We connected immediately. I was very weary of writing an endless string of papers suggesting better local and global policies for environmental conservation practices. My pilot light, my Russian-Italian passion flame, by now flickered very low as a result of over-thinking any number of problems. Yet this African earth mother gave me new clues on how to re-ignite it. She invited me to return to East Africa, to see how things really were on the ground, to put theory into practice—and to learn from her people.

And I couldn't help but answer her call.

MY GUIDE

Following the end of my first wildlife safari in Africa, I found myself at Gibb's Farm in Karatu, Tanzania, where I met with Ole Sululu, a Maasai born just a few kilometers away on the rim of Embakaai Crater in the Ngorongoro Conservation Area.

Sululu estimated that he was born in 1956, one of eleven children of the first wife of his father. Most of his full brothers and sisters—his father had seven wives—had chosen to leave their traditional Maasai village and pursue modern livelihoods as doctors, nurses, miners, and in positions in tourism and development. Many of his half-brothers and sisters, however, remained in the rural village. I wondered if his mother had encouraged her children to take up lives in the outside world, and it seemed that the entire extended family would certainly be an interesting study in the "nature versus nurture" debate. I asked Sululu about his journey from herding cattle as a boy to leading expensive, high-quality safaris up Mt. Kilimanjaro and into the Serengeti.

In almost perfect English he explained, "As a child, I stayed with a missionary from Europe in Ngorongoro who taught me the Western things—how to speak English, how to drive and cook. The missionary helped sponsor most of my brothers to go to school and sponsored me for tour guiding school, where I received a certificate that gave me the ticket to a job in the growing tourism industry in Arusha. Since 1980 I worked as a safari guide in Rwanda, Burundi, Tanzania, and Zaire, meeting people and seeing the land. It was a very challenging time because our culture was being disturbed. In the 1970s, there was a drought in my home area that led to a lot of cattle dying and people starving. So I was happy to get the opportunity to spend time with the missionary. It seemed better to start to think about getting out of the area at the time because there were no rains, no water, no food. There was no school there. The missionary gave me food and taught me a lot, a lot, a lot."

One day, when Sululu was grazing his father's cows, a vehicle drove by that seemed lost. It was a tourist group looking for Oldonyo Lengai--the Mountain of God, in the Maa language—and had taken a wrong turn. Sululu pointed out on the map where they were and in which direction they needed to go to reach their destination. The tour guide was very impressed with Sululu's map and English skills and asked him to come to town to interview for a job with their company. A month later, Sululu made the three-day walk to Arusha. He passed an exam with flying colors—knowing all the birds and wildlife species on the test, and his driving skills were excellent. "So, the company gave me a car to drive for groups, and that is how I started to work in tourism."

Sululu's full name is Lekoko Ole Sululu. Sululu is his surname and Ole means "son of" in Maa. The word "Sululu" literally translates as "swamp," and Sululu explained that it also means "hope," because a swamp "is a place that never comes dry," something vitally important in an arid land where people's wealth depends on the survival of their cattle. "Lekoko" means "son of grandmother"—a name he was given because children are often named after ancestors.

As we spoke, Sululu remembered how the missionary tried to teach Sululu and his people about Christianity. "That is what all the missionaries tried to do. They have this very strong religion. We just let them talk. And when they finished talking, we thought, okay, that is good. Many people in my village listened but never followed much of anything the missionaries said about religion."

Sululu remained drawn to the traditional way of the Maasai, moving in search of green pastures to graze their cattle. The traditional rhythm of life—grazing cattle, becoming a man through initiation, protecting the community—was wonderful, he said, a precious way of living. But as time marched on, it had become difficult to find good land on which to freely graze cattle. He knew that with climate change, more droughts could very possibly devastate the Maasai communities. And it was important for people to gain skills other than livestock raising.

I knew I was asking Sululu too many questions, but I was fascinated. He seemed to be a wonderful combination of bushman and modern Maasai. How was it possible for him to be both,

I asked. "I see many people who left our Maasai community to study in other parts of the world. And they have come back. They have kept their culture," he said.

From that first meeting, Sululu and I became great friends, and he ultimately became my guide on a decade-long psychological-spiritual journey. Over the years, our conversations about bridging indigenous and modern wisdom have never stopped. Together, we established a visionary organization that put into practice the concept of honoring traditional knowledge, while assisting communities to develop people's lives for the better—leading people-to-people safaris designed to share all we have discovered with travelers from the West.

Sululu is, in a very real sense, the co-author of this book. Many of its parables are results of experiences we shared together, inside Maasai villages and while traveling in the United States as well. He has listened to me for hours as I tried to make sense of the events I was experiencing, feeling many times as if my brain was unraveling, or as if I was looking up at my own culture from below and seeing its underbelly. Sululu has been as patient as a hartebeest as he has listened to thoughts coming from my often over-analytic mind. He has shared his insights with me, told me when he suspected I might be wrong about something, and has cheered me when I've made a breakthrough in understanding.

I know I have been blessed many times in my life, but it was a special blessing to meet Sululu and be invited by him to travel deep inside an indigenous culture, to have been accepted by his fellow tribespeople, the Maasai of East Africa, and to have learned some of their amazing ancient gems of wisdom. In return, I have made a promise to them to translate this rapidly disappearing knowledge into a form understandable to modern peoples; and to share this with my "tribe," whom the Maasai call "the paper people."

The Maasai don't do monologues. Ideas and plans emerge from inside of rich conversations. In fact, when you listen to a group of Maasai speaking together, it is as if they are singing, and the person speaking always receives assurance that his or her words matter. "Yes, we agree . . . right on, eh, eh."

In that spirit of Maasai sharing, here are some vignettes and conversations. Listen to how the gems of wisdom emerge through the singing.

Sululu on his mobile phone

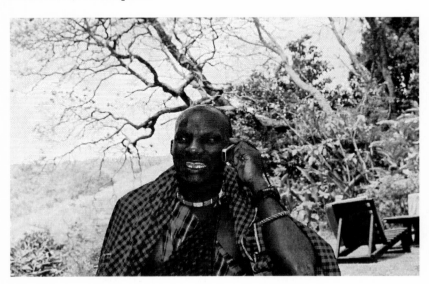

INTRODUCTION TO MAASAI COMMUNITY

The game drives in the renowned wildlife parks in Tanzania's
Northern Circuit ignited my mind with thoughts about environmental conservation in ways that were very different from how I
had considered the subject in graduate school. Wanting my eyes
to be as open as possible to new understandings, I had asked
my guides to bring me into the villages, to meet the people who
lived in and around the parks. At first they refused, telling me
that *mzungus*, white visitors, should not go to the villages because
there was too much poverty in them. But I insisted that I wanted
to truly see how the Tanzanian people lived—how the majority of
the people on this planet live—and eventually they consented and
took me to the villages.

I learned about community and wildlife conflicts and the ways
in which international organizations were working to distribute
more of the revenue earned from photographic and hunting safaris to the local people. I learned of the deforestation of indigenous
forests as people cut down more and more trees for fuel and to
make charcoal. I learned that the government of Tanzania was
unable to bring electricity in any form to the rural and even semi-
rural areas of the country, where eighty percent of its citizens live.

So many of the theories I had been teaching in my Environmental Sociology classes back home were sorely tested in real
time in East Africa, and I couldn't help but be moved by the
disparities between what I "knew" and what I now saw. Surely
there was a way I could help, I believed—some way in which I
could really get in there and support Tanzanian development, yet

maintain its incredible natural beauty. "Sustainable development" was the term of the moment in my professional circles, and I was certainly passionate about getting involved in the thick of it. But even with Sululu's help, I wondered if I could find my way in with respect, understanding, and compassion.

The answer, it turned out, was finding a way to connect with people on a spiritual level. During one of our game drives, my guide asked me what my religious denomination was. It seemed to be a common question among people in that region, heavily influenced by the work of Christian and Islamic missionaries. At first I chose not to answer, thinking the question was too personal to ask of a "stranger." But it wasn't inappropriate at all from his point of view. He persisted, and eventually I told him a few things about my background and beliefs.

In that case, he said, "You should visit my people, the Maasai. You will be like a sister to them," assuring me that they and I shared similar beliefs about a universal God or creator who can most easily be experienced in nature. Like virtually all indigenous peoples, the Maasai had a strong belief in the power of nature and its connection to the human spirit, he said.

According to Maasai oral history, their people originated from the area of Egypt, along the Nile River and migrated south through Sudan, Ethiopia, and Somalia around the fifteenth century, ultimately moving into Kenya and Tanzania between the seventeenth and late eighteenth centuries. It has always been challenging for the Maasai to maintain their traditional semi-nomadic pastoral lifestyle, no matter where they have traveled.

During my first visit to a Maasai homestead, I talked with

the people I met about health care, culture, medicine, and the natural environment, and I came away amazed. How could these people have such wisdom, without any formal education? I was overwhelmed, and I knew I clearly had something to learn from this community. In contrast to all the dancing around the edges of "what is wellness?" in America, the work I was doing with the alternative medicine boom, and in environmental conservation, I actually felt I was getting close to some *answers* here in the remote villages of East Africa. I wanted to learn more, and perhaps become a teacher and a student at the same time.

I was given a name, *Namelok*, meaning "Sweetie," a woman with a sweet heart. Unlike many of the previous researchers and international development workers who had come to their villages and asked many questions, I just sat and listened. And apparently the Maasai appreciated the difference. "When people asked you who you are," Sululu explained to me, "you spoke slowly, and from the heart. They believed you were very interested in them, open to hearing everything they said, not for any specific target. That is why they love you."

THE BIG EXCHANGE

We made a pact. I would help several Maasai communities address some of their most basic needs—poverty alleviation, clean water, modern education—and they would share with me the ways in which they healed their bodies, minds, and communities. The Maasai, like all indigenous communities I have spent time with, practice a giving and receiving cycle on a grand scale.

They engage in simple, short-term exchanges when someone trades a big bull for two heifers, yet they also enter into long-term agreements when one person agrees to donate cattle for a family member's wedding with the understanding that he will similarly be repaid years down the road. When you are part of a tight-knit community, this can be both a curse and a blessing, depending on how your own balance sheet adds up.

Fueled by my years learning about social and economic development, knowing what I knew about modern lifestyles in the West, and with new insights I had gained from Wangari, I was adamant about not simply responding to requests from the communities for boreholes, classrooms, and health clinics. I wanted to collaborate, to find a bridge between the good old ways and the good new ways.

If we were going to build classrooms, then we were going to provide computers with Internet access. If we were going to build health clinics, they were going to be based on integrated medicine. I found myself explaining that the West was not always best, while agreeing that some major improvements were necessary to help move people out of abject poverty.

In a Maasai community in Tanzania in 2001, we negotiated something along the following lines: the Maasai would teach me some of the secrets they had for maintaining emotional and spiritual wellbeing, and share with me the plant medicines they used for healing. In exchange, I would help them become more modern by building schools, cultivating medicinal plant nurseries, and connecting them to the world through information technology. I knew I had the experience, expertise and contacts, and that I could harness these resources to bring real change into the Maasai world. And I was passionate to learn what they had to teach me. It would be an extraordinary exchange—and it would transform my life.

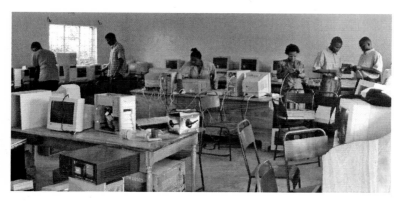

One of Terrawatu's first computer labs at a school in Tanzania, 2005

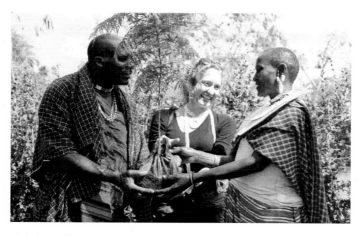

Sululu and I giving a plant to a women's network leader for their tree nursery in Mkonoo Village, Tanzania

KEEPING THE FIRE BURNING AT HEARTH AND HOME

Most of my friends and family were shocked that I actually planned to rent out my lovely home in Seattle and live virtually full-time in East Africa—and I was often surprised by their reactions. We all had spent so much time criticizing the current state of American society and talking about how unsatisfied we were to work longer and longer hours only to make more money to pay for the increasing cost of housing, health care, car maintenance, food, et cetera. I had made the decision to temporarily step off the national treadmill of production and consumption and check out another way of living, to be in a place that was just starting to be influenced by globalization, where people were hungry for American know-how. Didn't my Seattle friends think the idea was kind of cool?

I was committed, and it certainly seemed easier to close one file and open another, instead of trying to keep two lives going at the same time. Many people who have had a similar urge to expatriate and completely change their lives have sold all their worldly possessions and jumped ship to a new, completely different location. Yet it seemed right for me to be a bit less dramatic. I wanted to explore the landscape between two worlds, two cultures, and discover a bridge connecting them. Instead of the clash of civilizations, I wanted to choreograph the dance. It must have been the romantic Italian in me.

My friends kept the fire burning in my house in the village in Seattle over the years. The upstairs remained my bedroom, bath, and yoga room. When I returned occasionally, we would share the kitchen, dining room, and sitting room. We called it "the village house." When friends from East Africa came to visit, the doors to the unofficial "Tanzanian Embassy" would swing open and we would provide home-cooked meals of Pacific salmon, *nyama choma*, Swahili-style roast meat, polenta, an Italian version of *ugali*, the staple food of East Africa, and Maasai-style chai.

I combined foods and flavors of many regions of Tanzania, knowing the traditional food of the Maasai would not be too satisfying to my tribe in Seattle. I served both Italian and South African wine. And we would share stories—long conversations around the outdoor fire-pit that lasted long into the evening just as they did in Maasailand, stories about politics, economics, and family. I always felt I brought a piece of Africa with me when I returned to America. And I always enjoyed catching up with the current news and trends from the United States to take back with me to my villages in Africa. The Maasai have a word, *oloipung'o*, which means to travel away from your home and explore another piece of the world and then turn back and share it with your people. I loved the rewards of my *oliopung'o* experiences, and I shared them on both continents as bridges between the two.

Just prior to the collapse of the real estate market in the United States, I sold the village house in Seattle and downsized to a one bedroom flat in Miami, where the weather better suited my clothes and it was a slightly shorter hop across the pond. I still visit the village in Seattle, share African stories in person there when I can, and stay in close touch via the Internet. My mom now lives in southern California and always has a bed ready for me there. I carry my keys to my American home with me wherever I go, as a Maasai woman does when she sets out on safari. Knowing I have such special nests to fly to makes the whole *oloipung'o* experience more comfortable, and special.

MEDICINE FOR LIFE

This book began as one about the traditional medicine of the Maasai people in East Africa. But it ended up being a book about life. The information it contains was imparted to me largely via oral histories. I was fortunate to hear many, wonderful stories, and on the following pages I cull gems of wisdom most useful to us modern Westerners and weave them into parables familiar to us, stories that make it easy to understand how profound and timeless the indigenous ways are.

All indigenous cultures share similar worldviews. Known by some as "indigenous consciousness," this way of being in the world is innately holistic. Every individual is entirely woven into her natural environment; her mind and intellect shape and are shaped by those in her community. Her soul is the same soul as everyone else's; she simply wears her own costume while on earth during the time we know her physically.

Something that has fascinated me since back when I trained as an anthropologist and social psychologist is how science increasingly presents evidence that demonstrates the intrinsic value of what indigenous people have always known. Modern communities are springing up all over the globe that believe in universality, collective soul, and heart-lead businesses. Some people think this phenomenon means we are coming full circle, back to where we began. I think a better metaphor is a spiral, and that we are circling as we head higher up on an evolutionary flight. What remains constant is our connection as human beings to universal truths—verities I personally learned most clearly through working and living with the Maasai.

In many ways, my dozens of trips over a decade commuting from America to Tanzania were very much spiritual journeys. During the process, I learned amazing things about myself and my own ancestors. Living in such profoundly different environments allowed me to take a step out of both of them and have a bird's eye view of what was happening on the ground, and why. I became a witness to the sources of suffering in this world and could see why it is so difficult to alleviate. And, I learned from some beautiful earth-based people how to find health and happiness in some of the most unlikely places.

Tijing'u! Welcome inside!

2.

Daily Life

MORNING CHAI

Inosie olomoni (female, *engomoni*) *ilomon.*
Talk with your visitors, ask the news, and you all
will discover what is happening.

It was a particularly bad morning at the Starbucks. A couple of my
male friends had not "scored" with women they had been hunting
for some time. And, apparently, I was being blamed for jeopard-
izing one man's chances with another woman because I did not
speak glowingly enough about him in a recent chat with her. I was
back in Miami, one of my villages, and I treasure my morning coffee with my tribe, no matter how tense the mood.

"I am too rushed in the morning to sit down to drink tea," a
friend of mine named Simon complained. "Primitive societies
don't have to get their children ready for school, get dressed for
work, and commute long hours by car to the office."

"Actually, the Maasai do have a lot to prepare for in the

morning," I explained. "But they don't launch into the day until they open it properly over a cup of tea with their family and friends." Simon was not sure why I was making such a big deal about a simple cup of morning tea or coffee. So, I tried to describe how important I think it is to ritually open the day this way.

I told him I remembered one particular morning when I woke up in a Maasai home in a village in northern Tanzania, very close to the border with Kenya. Sululu and I had driven up from Arusha the night before to give our condolences to the family because the patriarch of the homestead recently had died. The deceased was a spiritual healer, an *olaiboni*, who had worked for years in that region, healing people with all kinds of diseases, both physical and emotional. People had come from all over northern Tanzania and neighboring Kenya to seek this man's assistance, and his passing was a huge loss to the community.

We had arrived the night before after driving off the main paved road for many kilometers in the dusty bush, passing giraffes and ostriches gracefully moving through the thorny acacia trees. After cracking open bottles of warm Kilimanjaro and Safari lagers, we talked with our hosts about what had happened to the *olaiboni*, who was still middle-aged. As I always did in those circumstances where the conversation rolled along in a mixture of Maa, Swahili, and a bit of English, I listened to the words I knew and comprehended as best I could by "reading through the lines" floating in the air. In ten years of living and working in indigenous communities in Africa, I have rarely felt that I completely missed what was being said or what was happening.

The *olaiboni*'s death was apparently being blamed on the conflict of spirits—spirits of Christian and Islamic origins—that had taken residence in his body, unknowingly to him, during a recent visit he made to the Swahili coast. It is a place known to be home to very powerful spirits that can confuse and lead to very dangerous consequences if one does not respect them. The healer may, in fact, have been "side-swiped," caught off guard because he had not properly protected himself. Long ago, I had learned not to dismiss talk like this as simply the worldview of "primitive peoples," uneducated in medical science and of using only spiritual language to describe physical life and death. Instead, I "translated" conversations by using concepts familiar to my own educational background and life experience, creating a kind of blend of indigenous and modern wisdom.

And this particular circumstance was quite significant. A highly-respected spiritual healer apparently had died because he had taken on the conflict between Christianity and Islam that was being played out on the ground in the region of the Swahili Coast, an area raw with incidents of terrorism between the two institutionalized religions. Some people claimed that the escalating level of violence in that region was caused by opposition to the U.S.-led wars in Afghanistan and Iraq, which were perceived as wars waged against Islam. Could conflicts in other regions of the world be connected to spiritual forces in Africa that eventually led to a healer's death? While I could imagine some plausible evidence to support such a link, I also knew the healer who had just passed away was overweight. Could his death, in fact, have been the result of undiagnosed diabetes or heart disease? The reality was the truth probably lay somewhere in between.

It was becoming clear that we were going to spend the night at the homestead. The sun had set, and because we had a small car problem during the drive to get there, it was probably best to not attempt to depart in the dark on a drive through a bush full of animals much larger and stronger than ourselves. The women showed me to a bed I could sleep in for the evening, and I was grateful. While I have spent my fair share of nights sleeping on cow skins in small mud dung huts, I am always happy to be offered a wood-frame bed with a foam mattress—simply because it means it will take me less time to sort out my back in the morning, less time spent in yoga postures and more time chatting over morning tea.

"Are you sure I can have this bed tonight?" I asked the mama of the homestead. "I know that I am displacing someone for the evening and always feel a bit bad about that."

"Of course," she replied, "you are the honored guest, traveling all this way to pay your respects to Babu." I must have been tired because after only a quick review of the events of the day and thinking briefly again about the death of the healer, I fell easily asleep.

I awoke to the sounds of morning in the boma, or homestead—cows, their bells clanking, being taken out to graze, children shouting as they began to play, birds greeting the day with song. I looked around at my surroundings to remind myself where I was, but the first thing I perceived was how I felt. How, I wondered, could I feel so calm and wonderfully at peace in such un-luxurious accommodations? The walls surrounding me were made of mud and dung plastered around pieces of timber. The floor was packed dirt. There was nothing else in the room other than the bed and a chair made of bamboo and goatskin on which I had put my small bag the night before. No bedside lamp, no electricity. All I knew was that I felt at ease and fresh, like a brand new day had dawned and all the complexity of the day before had been magically washed away. Had these people *done something* to me while I slept? I later realized that they had. My Maasai hosts had simply enveloped me in a vital aspect of their culture, in this case the collective belief in properly closing one day and resting before beginning afresh the next.

I described to my friend Simon how then I had taken a short walk in the soft morning light, taking in the sights and smells of the bush—flat-topped acacia trees seeming to support the sky, the dry red earth, ancient and raw, which would become heavy, un-navigable mud with the first of the big rains. It was almost impossible not to feel the earth breathe there, I told him.

"But Tanya, most people don't live in such an environment anymore. We walk down urban sidewalks to our local café."

"Of course," I said that morning in Miami, "it is certainly challenging to find peace walking through traffic-filled and polluted streets, but it doesn't mean it is not possible." I've done it in Mumbai, a booming, hectic city in the country that gave birth to yoga and strategies for finding inner calm. It is not so much about what is outside rather than what is inside. "You can still maintain that fresh morning mind," I explained, "starting your day's drive in a bright and easy manner instead of immediately slamming it into high gear and speeding down the highway. Everybody has their own way of waking up to the day, and each day is different.

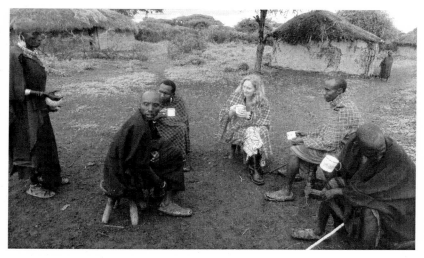

Morning chai in Maasailand, sitting on tri-pod stools

All I am saying is that it is somehow good to do your own rituals that inspire you to launch off into the day with joy and wonder."

As I returned from my walk people had begun to bring three-legged stools carved out of single logs outside so we could enjoy our morning chai in the crisp African air. There was not a lot of talking yet, but we all greeted each other and asked the almost universal question. *Itudumunye?* "How did you wake up?" It's a simple inquiry I love, because I always get the distinct sense that the person asking truly wants to know, curious whether her experience is similar to yours. It is a gauging kind of question, one that allows you to work out the general feeling of the morning, and whether it will be a peaceful, uneasy, or perhaps celebratory day.

Morning conversation over tea in Maasailand is a ritual called *ilomon*, and it's not only important for generating a kind of consensus about the day ahead and assigning people's tasks in the process. It also always includes some discussion about the dreams people had during the night. The Maasai attach a lot of meaning to dreams, especially because they often warn of threats to the all-important livestock and to the community as a whole.

"It is really not that different than our meetings at the coffee shop in the morning. I just don't think we are aware of it as much as we could be."

"What do you mean?" Simon asked.

"Well, if you really listen to the conversations people are having at breakfast tables and in coffee shops around America, they are sorting out their roles in their families and villages. After all, you have spent the night in your own world, even if you are sleeping next to somebody, it is still just you and the people and events in your dreams, if you are lucky to see them or remember them. So when the "real" day begins, as social animals we need to belong, to re-enter our place in the universe. Unfortunately, many people end up talking about their own experiences of the morning and what they have to do that day without too much emphasis on how we are all in it together."

"Well, that's because we focus on ourselves first," my friend in Miami reminded me.

"Yes, and that's important, but it is not an either/or thing. You are who you are because of your relationship with others. That's a classic African worldview, popularized by the Zulu word *ubuntu* that Desmond Tutu and Nelson Mandela used in their inspirational talks. The Maasai embrace it wholeheartedly. It is really lovely, because this way of being in the world is so much less stressful. You know, whether the ship sinks or sails along is not because of any one person, we are all sailing together. Too much emphasis on ME so often leads to unnecessary stress, as if the weight of the whole world is on each of our shoulders."

"What about the people who rush out of the house without having a conversation with anyone and picking up their coffee at the drive-thru?" Simon wanted to know.

"Well, it's just going to take them that much longer to start up their engine to flow through the day, regardless of the number of espresso shots in their cappuccino."

"You know, Tanya, not everybody thinks about 'who am I?' and 'what's my place in the world?' when they first wake up in the morning," Simon laughed.

"No, of course not. Not consciously at least. But it sure helps to have some sense of meaning, otherwise what's the point?" I said. "You can see the people who are swimming aimlessly along. Their faces look tired. Their bodies look tired."

My memory took me back to Africa and the countless mornings I held a tin cup of chai tightly to warm my hands. I sipped the rich tea made with fresh cow's milk boiled with black tea, and medicinal roots and leaves of plants that boost the immune system. Very efficient, I always thought, to combine the multi-vitamin with one's morning beverage—species that included *oloisuki* (*Zanthoxylum chalybeum*), *olamuriaki*, (*Carissa edulis*), and *ormangulai*, all of which help the body build antibodies and fight off disease. With a bit of sugar to sweeten the bitter taste of the herbs, it was like drinking the earth, and it was directly nourishing me.

On the morning that I was describing for Simon, I learned over chai that everyone awakened with a peaceful feeling in the Maasai *boma*. People clearly appreciated the fact that Sululu and I had made the effort to visit and pay our respects to the departed healer. The discussion we had the night before about the cause or causes of his death had been helpful to everyone. We cleared some air and everyone awakened more refreshed. There was a lovely buoyancy to the morning—and even more smiles and laughter than usual.

"I think I'm beginning to understand what you mean about this morning chai ritual," Simon offered. "I kept getting hung up on the word ritual. I tend to think of ritual in the negative, like something that we *have* to do but don't want to do. What you're saying is that it really is a simple activity that is full up with meaning that just makes people feel good."

"Yep, you got it exactly," I told him. "In the States, we tend to do these things only on special occasions, like weddings and graduations. You know, the staging of bachelor and bachelorette parties and dinners with toasts and speeches about how the persons being honored are beginning a new stage in their life and the effect that has on the whole community."

"And what you're saying is that you can create this feeling of meaning and belongingness in even simple activities, like morning coffee."

"In anything, really. It is not so much the behavior itself, but rather the awareness of whatever it is you are doing is guided by something larger than your own individual mind and body. A universal force that reminds us that we are all in this together. So comforting, so very tribal."

SUGGESTED PRACTICE

Take a moment to reflect on your day. How did you wake up? What did you do to move yourself from solitary sleep to engaging yourself with other people?

How did you feel when you began to engage with other people? How do you feel now?

Are there ways you can be more conscious about your morning activities that may make you feel more connected to others in your life? What would these be?

Set an intention to connect yourself more deeply to your tribe for one week and see how you feel. Write down your thoughts and feelings when they arise.

RECIPE FOR MORNING CHAI

A way to begin each day, modern Maasai-style: fill a small pot half full of water and heat it. Add a half teaspoon of good black tea leaves for each cup of tea you are making. Add a healthy sprinkling of spices. The best way to do this is to keep an airtight container full of the following spice mix: small pieces of cinnamon stick, dried orange peel, ground dried ginger, coriander, cardamom seeds [removed from their pods], cloves, and black peppercorns, all mashed up a bit with a mortar and pestle. Experiment with the proportions of each until you get your favorite blend.

Heat all this until it boils. Now, you can add pieces of medicinal plant bark and roots. In Tanzania we use *oloisuki* (*Zanthoxylum chalybeum*), and *olesupeni* (*Helinus integrifolius*) to strengthen the body, increase immunity levels, and treat back pain. Boil for another minute. Now, add whole milk until the chai becomes a nice, light beige color, then lower the heat. Just before the liquid comes to a boil again, pour it through a strainer into a thermos. You can place a small strainer on a funnel to make this process easier.

Place the thermos out on a table with cups and teaspoons. Serve with brown sugar or honey, so your morning chai ritual companions can sweeten the tea in the way they like.

While chai can be a meal in itself, if you are really hungry, serve with *chapati*. We also like to place a plate of fruits nearby; mangos, Asian apple-pears, and red bananas are a favorite in Tanzania.

Make sure the first thing you put in your mouth in the morning is warm. Drinking cold juice or even water out of the refrigerator can alter your body temperature and therefore make the chai taste strange—as well as jar your stomach! Sit around the table and enjoy the blessings of good chai and your morning companions. In Africa, we often talk about the dreams we had the night before, then our hopes for what we want to accomplish during this new day. Once the thermos is empty, it is time to head to the office or begin household tasks.

Of course, if you made too much chai, it is great to take the thermos with you and enjoy a late morning cup. If your morning chai companions are not under your roof, schedule a connection call over the phone or Internet while you both "virtually" enjoy your cups of warm beverage together.

FOOD

On another splendid morning in East Africa, I climbed out of my tent just after dawn and walked through the bush that encircled the Maasai family's homestead where I was staying. I needed to use the loo, in this case a simple hole in the earth overlooking the extraordinary landscape of the Great Rift Valley. It had to be the best view from a loo in the world, I thought to myself.

As I was walking back to my tent, my ears caught the sound of

The Great Rift Valley photographed from Monduli, Tanzania

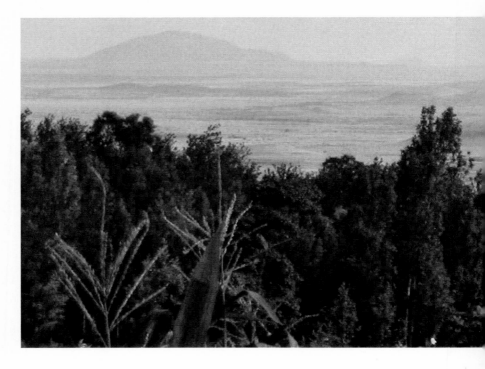

clanging bells. It was time to take the cattle out to graze. It was a sound I loved, one that seemed to me to be the music of pure pastoralism, and it was an infinitely more peaceful noise than a morning commute to the office in most major cities around the world. Many aspects of a pastoral nomadic lifestyle are truly blessings.

Because they subsist on livestock, the traditional Maasai diet is comprised of milk and meat. When I first arrived in Tanzania, I found it truly puzzling how people with such amazing physiques and energy could live on such a basic diet. No fruits or vegetables?

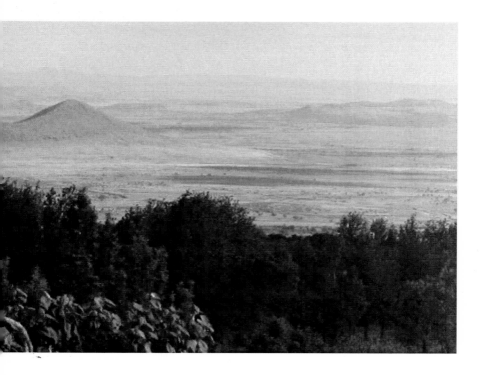

Surely they had to be malnourished. As I learned more about their daily lifestyle, the integral role of livestock in their lives, and how the Maasai nourish themselves not only with their cows, goats, and sheep, but also with native plants, I discovered that this is a diet they very consciously chose. For centuries, the Maasai have had contact with agriculturalists, and sporadically have added grains, vegetables, and other crops to their diets, but the majority still prefer subsisting on milk and meat—and blood—whenever possible.

Maasailand is a rough place. For much of the year, the hot African sun beats down strongly on the land. Grasses are hardy; trees and plants are able to withstand severe heat and long periods of drought. Large vegetarian wildlife such as giraffes and elephants roam widely, chopping away at the leaves and fruits of many plants, sometimes stripping them bare. When the rains arrive, the world becomes green and lush and the cows receive their greatest gift—the green grass which they in turn convert to muscle and to meat. It's a season, Sululu explained, that the Maasai have come to call "Christmas."

I have never been a big meat eater, and have been completely vegetarian during long stretches of my life—especially when I have lived in places where the source of the available meat was not clear or, when I knew animals had been fed chemical supplements before they were slaughtered. But when I lived in Maasailand I did, of course, eat meat. It was all there was to eat. I knew the animals it had come from were healthy, but most importantly, I ate it because I was offered it by my Maasai friends. Knowing how hard they worked grazing their livestock—traveling for months at a time in search of green pastures—and what big a sacrifice it is for them to ultimately slaughter one of the herd, I was always full of respect and appreciation.

The Maasai don't eat meat every day. Milk is the true staple. Milk, rather than water, is used to boil the tea and medicinal roots and bark for morning chai, and is consumed throughout the day as well. Children often eat a porridge made from boiled milk and ground maize. And milk that has sat for some hours or days, called "sleeping milk," is consumed as a drinkable yogurt. Traditionally, the Maasai consumed meat only about once a week, and that often remains the case today. But when they do eat meat, they *eat meat*. Consuming massive quantities of beef or mutton or goat at a single sitting allows their bodies to store the calories the meat provides, and traditionally they have consumed a medicinal soup with the meat that promotes their digestion and helps them expel non-nourishing parts of the meat while converting the rest into energy.

I remember my first visit to Sululu's father's *boma* in Embakaai. I was doing research in Maasailand for the United Nations Development Program (UNDP) and had spent many days and nights in traditional homesteads, so I knew what to plan for. I had wisely taken home with me the remaining Indian food I had ordered at a restaurant in Arusha the night before. And I packed fresh fruits and nuts in our vehicle, along with plenty of water. The journey took all day as we passed through beautiful lands teaming with wildlife and rarely seen by tourists.

When we arrived at the homestead, it was early evening, not too long before the sun would set. Sululu and I were greeted very warmly, with much singing and dancing by the women of the village. We then sat down with the men to share some beer and catch up on the news of the family and village. As always, "Dr. Tanya" was allowed to sit with the men, and Sululu would translate the parts of the conversation I did not understand. At one point, I realized I was *very* hungry. I knew some of the warriors had been told by his father to slaughter a goat in our honor, but I also knew that building a proper fire and roasting the meat was going to take a while.

I asked Sululu if it would be all right if I got the Indian food from the car. He said yes, but explained that I would have to take it to the women's dwelling and eat it there. The Italian in me immediately wanted to object—dinner should be eaten with family and friends, with lots of talking between bites. My American feminist side wanted to make clear that a woman can do whatever she chooses to do, and if I wanted to eat in front of the beer-drinking men, then who was going to stop me?

But another voice silenced me, and I quietly walked to the women's dwelling, where a sweet woman who was a member of Sululu's extended family—he has more than thirty sisters— showed me where I could sit and eat. Maasai men eat roughly, often crunching into bones and polishing off every morsel of meat and bit of marrow. They do not like women to see them eating in this way, so therefore, men and women have always eaten separately, in traditional settings.

My guide left me alone to go back to the group of ladies she had been speaking with, and I could tell she had no interest in sharing my lentils, spinach, paneer, and naan. I sat alone in a dark hut and savored my food in silence. While I had eaten many a meal by myself when I was traveling alone, this was different. Those meals were typically in restaurants with others around me, and I was often reading a book or magazine. This time, it was just me and my food, with an entire extended family outside making sure I was happy and getting what I needed—at least to the degree they could understand. As Sululu explained, people like me who eat "grass" seem very odd to them.

I was comfortable eating alone, and it felt special to eat in a place that is sacred for women. I think this moment was honestly the first time I ever *felt* my food—aware that an external substance was going into my body and nourishing me. I remember feeling full quite quickly. And I even saved a bit of Indian food for later, just in case. It is amazing how something you do so habitually—like eating—can change when you do it with awareness.

Years later, I spent some days at an ashram in India and was required to eat in silence. In that place, I was surrounded by hundreds of people sitting on the floor using their hands to scoop up lentils, and at each meal while I was there I remembered my time in the women's hut in Embaakai.

SUGGESTED PRACTICE

If you eat meat, consider eating meat only from animals you have raised yourself or from people you know.

Eat only when you are truly hungry. Say a blessing of appreciation before you take a bite, either silently or out loud.

Try eating only with men if you are a man and with women if you are a woman. Notice how it feels.

Practice eating a meal in silence. Stay aware of the whole process. How do you experience this?

SULULU IN SEATTLE

It was not easy to get Sululu to drive with me to the Whole Foods Market in Seattle. I told him we needed to get some things to make dinner for my friends that evening. Going to the market was women's work, he said. I explained that in the United States both men and women shopped for food. Plus, I wanted to show him a modern American supermarket.

I parked the car in an underground garage and we took an elevator up to the market. Needless to say, his experience of Whole Foods was vastly different than walking around the local market in Arusha, chatting with the women selling fruits and vegetables.

We discussed what to make for my friends, who were eager to try "Africa food." We settled on roast chicken, polenta (the closest thing you can get to *ugali*, an East African staple food made of ground maize) and some vegetables. In the vegetable section, I chose some green beans, carrots, potatoes and mushrooms. Sululu was curious. "Who do you speak to about the price you will get those for?" When I explained the price was fixed and based on weight, and a machine would weigh the bags at checkout and determine the price, he shot me a look of astonishment.

When we walked up to a long glass case filled with chicken parts—legs, breasts, skinless, boneless—he wondered where the *chickens* were, and was shocked by the prices. I explained they were free-range, organic chickens—the closest we could find to the Tanzanian chickens he was accustomed to, but this concept seemed to confuse him even more. A good chicken at home would cost only a tiny fraction of the Whole Foods price.

I knew Sululu likes cheese, having spent some time in Holland. In the cheese section, a woman behind the cheese counter let him try some different cheeses from Europe, but when he tried to barter down the price, he couldn't understand why she simply refused. I could feel his energy dropping; he was getting overwhelmed, and I knew we should be leaving soon.

Before we departed, I asked if he would like to see the traditional medicine section. "But where's the medicine?" he asked when I showed him rows of carefully packaged offerings—capsules in white plastic containers and tinctures in little glass bottles. Where were the bark, roots, leaves and other parts of plants that a traditional doctor uses when working with a patient? I explained about processing, standardization, and marketing, but it didn't make sense to him. Nor could he understand why a doctor wasn't present to dispense these "medicines." So, I showed him a touch-screen computer shoppers could use to enter symptoms and get recommendations for what type of herbal remedy to try.

"Why has your culture replaced people with machines?" Sululu asked—a question I opted to try to answer another time. When we got back home, Sululu was happy to help prepare our meal. Having been a safari guide for years, at least he was accustomed to seeing men in a kitchen, and had even done some cooking himself. Because Maasai men always do the roasting of the meat, I figured I was on safe ground by giving him that task. We were going to use an oven instead of an open fire, I explained. I then went upstairs to take a shower.

Half an hour later, as I was descending the stairs, I heard a loud noise coming from the kitchen. As I rushed in, there was Sululu, hacking away at the chicken, explaining that he was cutting the chicken into pieces so that it would cook faster in the cooking machine.

I was exasperated. "But we could have bought the chicken in pieces to begin with!"

"But Dada, I needed to see the whole chicken. Otherwise, how do we trust where those pieces come from?" I thought he had a good point.

SUGGESTED PRACTICE

Enjoy the conveniences we have today by walking through a modern supermarket chatting and discussing food choices with a good friend or family member. Appreciate where your food comes from.

Continue the conversation in the kitchen. So much more enjoyable than popping a frozen meal into a microwave, make cooking a sacred part of the day. Does your food taste different when you place your attention on the whole process?

Consider shopping for food at your local farmer's market, or fish and meat market. Many of the providers are regulars, and you can get to know each other over time. Find out what is in season and where your food is coming from that day.

RAISING THE LIVESTOCK BANK

Ore engata na ingishu.
Time is cattle, every time is cattle time,
time to take care of the cattle.

I always find it beautiful to watch young Maasai boys herding large groups of cattle through the savannah lands in search of green grass and water. Dressed in their red shukas, they walk determinedly through the different hues of brown coloring the savannah. These boys have a big responsibility at a young age. They are guarding and caring for their family's livestock, its food supply, and its bank—all standing on four hooves.

Maasai boys herding cattle, Sinya, Tanzania

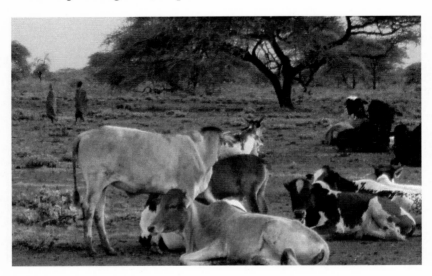

Cows are everything for the Maasai. Every member of a Maasai family contributes to the health and size of the livestock. Mothers prepare morning chai for their sons before they head out to graze the herd so the boys do not get too hungry. The cows, goats, and sheep technically "belong" to the male head of household, but everyone plays a role in their care.

There are always at least two older sons—ranked as warriors—protecting the perimeters of the grazing cows. They stay as much as a kilometer away from the grazing livestock and guard against potential thieves and hungry wild animals. Fathers scout out where the grasses are greener and water holes are full, and glean information in conversations with other male heads of household on local market days. Wives and daughters awaken early every day to milk the cows before they are taken out to graze. When anyone notices that a cow is ill, everyone comes together to help cure the animal and prevent the disease from spreading. When the cows are happy, the family is happy.

For most people living in modern societies, the goal of work is to make money to support yourself and your family. Like the Maasai, those of us on the frontline of income generation are supported by family members and friends who contribute resources—logistical and emotional—that allow us to do what we do. Unfortunately, we are not often as aware of being part of this "workforce" as we can be, and therefore do not appreciate everything that's required to increase our bank accounts.

I have often watched young Maasai boys in their classic balancing pose—standing with one foot on the earth and the other resting against their thigh as they watch their cattle eat grass and drink water. It is striking how much time it takes for these two fundamental activities to occur, and how dependent everyone is on the climate and rains. In a related way, in the modern information economy many of us spend a great deal of time talking, writing, and convincing others to consume what it is we are offering. These offerings are highly dependent on the rapidly changing climate of opinion. Time has become our most precious commodity, as it always has been. For us, time is money. For the Maasai, time is cows.

WORSHIPPING NATURE

During a visit to Embaakai, Sululu's birthplace, we went for a walk to the local village at the base of Kerimasi Mountain. The path we took edged from the crater rim along the escarpment and provided us with truly stunning views. I felt like I was in an airplane as I looked down on the Ngorongoro Conservation Area with its heavily forested land and wide craters. *Oldonyo Lengai*, the "Mountain of God," an active volcano, was visible in the center of the Rift Valley escarpment. Cape buffalo, zebra, and wildebeest grazed in the distance as we walked toward the village of Engovironi.

At one point we noticed a small concrete structure with a tin roof standing exposed to the mid-day sun. It had no windows and its interior had to be brutally hot. As we got closer, Sululu noticed a cross on the front side of the building. He asked a Maasai warrior who walked up to us the denomination of the little church. The young man looked at the building, then back at us and said, *Mikiyolo*. "We have no idea, nobody has ever been inside." He then opened his arms as if to embrace the view of the land laid out at our feet and continued, "Why would you go inside that place when you have this?"

I joined him in looking at our surroundings, and the innate beauty of the place took my breath away. He was right: it was a very special place in which to pray and count one's blessings— and it sure beat baking inside a concrete and tin-roofed church.

RHYTHM OF THE DAY

After a breakfast of morning chai and discussion about what needed to be done in the community that day, traditional Maasai days unfolded rhythmically. In the years before schools were built, young boys herded cattle and girls helped their mothers collect water and firewood, as well as milk the cows and goats. Men often sat together to plan the future and talk about family matters. Sometimes men, and occasionally women, would walk to neighboring villages for meetings, circumcision ceremonies, and other events that marked rites of passage, visits that could take days or weeks depending on the distances traveled and time needed to accomplish tasks or sort through issues.

By early evening, cows, goats, and sheep would be brought back to their corral and mothers and girls would milk them again as soon as they returned. If ground maize was available, some of the milk would be used to make porridge. If it was not, the milk would be drunk for dinner. Depending on supply, a few times a week meat would be roasted and eaten with great ritual, the women and children eating separately from the men.

People would go to sleep early, unless there was something

important to discuss—and when I was present at a Maasai *boma* for either a project or a personal visit, there was inevitably something to discuss. I relished the sharing of ideas that seemed to flow so freely without a specific agenda, power points emerging through the ebb and flow of the conversation. On many occasions, the talking would come to a close and be replaced with singing— particularly when the lyrics of a traditional song seemed to capture a truth about what we had been discussing.

With the advent of schools, things have changed. Although families remain close-knit, choices now have to be made about who performs traditional daily activities. While sending a child to school is now a government requirement, in many parts of Maasailand the benefits of this "new" form of education are not yet clear to people. A great deal of the work that our organization, Terrawatu, has been engaged in over the years attempts to tackle this issue. How can Maasai communities receive benefits from modern education and still maintain the traditional aspects of their culture that keep them strong and healthy?

It is important to realize that in the daily life of the Maasai, the waking state of consciousness is only one level of the day. A companion dreaming state of consciousness is equally real and vital. As Sululu explained to me, when an important question is asked of a Maasai, he or she seldom answers immediately. A wise man or woman will always say, *Alo airagie ina.* "I will sleep on that."

The more time I spent with the Maasai, the more I found them to be the most pragmatic spiritual people I had ever met. The warriors, elders, and medicine women I got to know would move effortlessly between grounded practicality, their dreams, and the transcendental realm of being, by which I mean being a witness to your own self. I know it sounds romantic, but despite the rough conditions in rural Maasai *bomas*, I virtually always felt and experienced a profound depth and richness in human connection and conversation, both with words and without.

LIFE HAS SEASONS

Ingataitiin olari.
Life has seasons, things change,
be patient, things will change.

The Maasai calendar is demarcated by the moon cycle and climate changes. When I first started working in Maasailand, I scheduled a meeting for the first day of the month. I remember diligently putting together an agenda and preparing my materials for a meeting on February 1st.

After waiting hours for my transport when the day arrived, I finally asked, "What happened to our meeting plan?"

"The meeting is the beginning of the month, not today," Sululu responded, and I did not understand. He explained that the beginning of the month wouldn't arrive until the first sliver of the new moon first appeared in the sky. Silly me. I downloaded a moon calendar on my laptop and never made that mistake again.

Given the moon's natural cycles, there *are* twelve months in the Maasai calendar, just like ours. Each month is described by the amount of rainfall that is typically received during that time. The Maasai calendar can be complicated and confusing, because different parts of the region receive different amounts of rainfall. Yet there are generally three seasons: the season of long rains, the drizzle season, and the season of short rains. Each month within the season is labeled by the expected weather. For example, *oladalu* is a time that is normally hot, dry, and sunny. During *oenioing'ok*, bulls normally become fierce from the scarcity of food and water. They have to be tied and left at home, because otherwise the bulls would drive the herd home too early. During *kushin*, small white and black birds appear that feed in the midst of the cattle. At *pushuka*, certain herbs ripen, many trees shed their leaves, and flowers bloom.

It goes without saying that life in the bush requires traditional Maasai to "live in harmony with nature." When temperatures drop in higher elevations, women keep their fires burning all day and people stay inside their homes as much as possible. When it is too hot, people rest in the shade of trees and move at a slower pace. When the first of the rains come, there are celebrations throughout Maasailand. Women milk the cows and bring containers of milk to neighboring *bomas* where warriors come out to drink and girls sing together. It is a time for sharing the wealth.

Just because we have developed methods to live our daily lives in almost the same way every day, with very little seasonal variation, does not mean it is a harmonious way of living for body, mind, or spirit. In fact, simply responding mindfully to the reality of the day's weather can help us make food and activity choices that connect us to natural cycles and the flow of the seasons. Healthier and happier lifestyles are the outcomes of rhythmic and fluid days, weeks, and months.

SUGGESTED PRACTICE

Honor the changes you observe in the natural environment. Your body will need more energy to stay warm during the cold season. Eat, sleep, and work differently.

If you live in a cooler and wet climate, celebrate the days when the sun comes out. If you live in a hot and sunny climate, celebrate the cleansing rain.

3.

Knowing Yourself

MAKING A PLAN

I focused my first few months in Tanzania on my own search
to find a way to make a useful contribution. But I did not easily
fit into the already well-established organizations and programs
dedicated to making a difference in Africa—the Peace Corps,
Medicens sans Frontiers (Doctors without Borders), the United
Nations Development Program (UNDP), and others.

With my level of education and commitment to working at
the grassroots, learning as I taught, I did not want to reinvent the
wheel, but rather repair or add some spokes. I wanted to cultivate
a perspective and strategies that I could use to inform and consult
with program officers, many of whom spent their days in offices
far away from the villages.

I did not hope to "save Africa." That naïveté went by the way-
side early in my studies of political sociology and social change,
and from what I quickly understood as soon as I was immersed in
Maasai communities in Tanzania. In fact, one Maasai elder once

suggested to me, "Namelok, perhaps with what we teach you, you can go and save America!"

I often found myself reflecting on the simple life of the Maasai, with its profound practicality and resourcefulness. Because their cows are at once their source of food and their money, this critical resource has to constantly have good grass to graze—grass that must never be destroyed by overgrazing. No one cares more about protecting and sustaining grasslands in Africa than the Maasai.

Sululu and the people to whom he introduced me showed me great respect from the outset and offered me the opportunity of a lifetime—one that would add to all of my years of American education and virtually countless hours of academic investigation into my field—the chance to put visions into action. I felt a bit apprehensive. Could I do this? Something was niggling at me deep down. I recognized that a childish part of me needed to grow up, fast.

I needed good advice on how to create this position for myself in the Maasai community. It was going to take a level of confidence, creativity, and resource mobilization that I had never had to draw on before. So, I briefly returned to Seattle and called on a traditional healer who was originally from Nigeria. In less than two months of working together a way forward appeared, although the process of discovery was not easy.

Deep and important revelations about my personal history had to be uncovered, sorted and cleansed so that a new "Tanya" could appear, and the Nigerian healer introduced me to the world of indigenous spirit healing firsthand. I endured a series of rituals based on those used by the Igbo people of Nigeria to initiate tribal members into adulthood. At thirty-one, I had thought I was an adult already, but with the healer's help I realized that modern Americans hold many beliefs that prolong adolescence, and with it, create a certain fear of readily acting on one's convictions. Young Americans like me talked a lot, he helped me understand, but few were ready to put our money and actions where our mouths were.

The entirety of the initiation process is rather difficult to describe, yet the ways in which I was transformed amaze me to this day. The healer instructed me, for example, to email as little as possible during the initiation. Email was originally intended as a tool to facilitate communication, especially between people who are geographically distant. It has done this, but it has also encouraged people—friends, lovers, bosses—to shy away from facing each other and saying what they really mean. I realized that I had been spending huge amounts of time typing email messages intended to help others heal from relationship ills, solve problems with their jobs, and even contribute to global environmental policy with colleagues. Words and emotions were spilling all over my keyboard, but because they were never contained in a serious, intentionally sacred space, few problems were properly addressed nor solved in ways they could have been.

Indigenous models for problem-solving involve holding meetings face-to-face, under a sacred tree, with everyone talking openly and sincerely about what he or she has experienced or perceived. Only those who can contribute—who need to be there—are invited to the meeting. Problems get worked through from all angles, and sometimes take a long time to solve. In modern societies, in contrast, with constant input of information, issues, and ideas, it is easy for us to lose our concentration. A problem may be important to us, but so are many others. We have a hard time following things through with intention and attention.

So, I stopped emailing, limiting my typing to emergency correspondence. I needed to conserve my energy, work on my own issues, and cultivate a new pathway for myself. I love my friends and family but they needed to wait until I could really be there for them, strong and clear about myself and my purpose.

LEARNING TO SEE THE PLAN

After I returned to Seattle from my first trip to Tanzania, I had encountered several women born in Africa who echoed a similar idea to me, suggesting I rewind the video of my life and watch the scenes again, this time looking for an underlying plot. When I did this, I immediately saw why I had chosen an anthropology-sociology major in university and studied sociology and social psychology in graduate school. It was because I had an innate fascination with how the movements of the universe affect the individual, and vice versa. I had also unconsciously taken the baton from my late father, a man fascinated by pharmacy and healing, and began to move toward uncovering indigenous origins of mind-body-spirit wellness in ways in which he would have approved.

To help me gain confidence about the plot of my life, I spent a great deal of time reflecting, meditating, and journaling during my work with the traditional healer. Eventually I sketched a plan that I knew was the right one. The specific details of what, where, and how I was going to live and work needed to be defined, but I had painted the broad strokes. I would have two home-bases, one in Africa and one in America. This was both unusual and essential.

I knew too many people who left a place where they lived out of anger at their inability to resolve issues, often making it difficult to ever return. I didn't want to burn bridges; I wanted to create them. I needed a strong U.S. home village to support me, especially because I would also be living and working in a place very distant and different. My plan involved putting resources where my mouth was and organizing a group of people who would undertake authentic, grassroots development projects. I also committed to sharing what I would learn in Africa with fellow tribespeople in America who, like me, were eager to work productively in the international arena.

I still had no idea where to begin, but the traditional healer told me simply to watch for signs. Yet where? My usual flood of emails had dried to a small trickle since I had stopped writing them. Phone calls had become scarcer as I had detached myself from most of the web of activity in my old life and found my way forward. I kept reading literature on environmental degradation, globalization, and world trade, hoping to find a slot into which I could fit.

About a week after announcing my new plan to a few friends in Seattle in a small ceremony held at my home in Greenlake, I received a short email from an old colleague I had not heard from in a while. It was a "charged" message, the kind that makes you stop for a moment because you sense its importance as it arrives. The message was from a professor at Princeton; we had been good friends when she was a post-doc at the University of Washington. She was a fellow environmentalist and social scientist who seriously wanted to make a difference in the world. It read simply, "Don't know what you are up to these days but I may have something you would be interested in. Can we set up a phone date? Let me know."

When we spoke on the phone a couple of days later, she said she had received my Christmas card with a photo of me on top of Mt. Kilimanjaro. At the time, she was actively looking for some-one to help her with her consultancy at the MacArthur Founda-tion on a project investigating the impact of human migration patterns on coastal ecosystems in Asia and Africa. As a specialist in human migration and demography, she knew very little about fisheries issues, but I appeared to her in a dream the night after she received my card, and she awakened with the memory of my Ph.D. research on salmon in the Pacific Northwest.

Yes! Of course, I wanted to help, I said. Yes, I could fly to Washington, D.C. the following week to help moderate a panel at an American Association for the Advancement of Science (AAAS) meeting. Yes, I would love to travel to Penang, Malaysia in a month to meet the international researchers involved in the project. I did not know where it all would lead, but it was certainly a door I was willing to walk through. I knew it would lead me to the place I was meant to go next.

The MacArthur project was fascinating. I did what I could to help the research teams' important findings get published in a journal that people would read. And, I met wonderful people, like-minded folks who truly were excited about working in the interna-tional development arena. My professional passions were ignited.

One member of the consulting team worked for the Global Environmental Facility (GEF) in Washington. She liked the ideas I

shared with her about development and asked if I was interested in
submitting a proposal for a project that would be funded through
her facility by monies received from the World Bank, UNDP, and
UNEP. I explained what I really wanted to do was employ the strategies of Wangari Maathai's Green Belt Movement in working with
the Maasai people of Tanzania to conserve their traditional medicine and indigenous healing knowledge. And, I explained, I wanted
to share the project activities with fellow Americans who were
interested in joining me in this "earth work."

"Perfect!" she replied. "Preserving traditional medicine is
hot right now from the GEF perspective, and anybody who can
truly work with the Maasai can get support." She did caution that
bringing along other Americans was beyond the scope of her
organization, but I knew I could find another way to do that.

So, I began working on a proposal. But it was difficult to write
from my desk in Seattle. I needed to know more about the issues
in Maasailand in Tanzania than what I had learned from my brief
visit seven months earlier. I needed more information than what
I could read about in the library or online. I needed to get back to
East Africa.

A month before I was scheduled to meet with my contact at
GEF at a meeting in Vienna, I read an online posting for the "First
Regional Conference on Medicinal Plants, Traditional Medicines
and Local Communities in Africa." It would be held in Nairobi,
Kenya in conjunction with the Fifth Meeting of the Conference
of the Parties (COP-5) of the Convention on Biological Diversity
(CBD). There were always countless postings about meetings and
conferences, but this one looked truly interesting.

I quickly wrote an abstract about a talk I could give on using African healing knowledge to treat chronic western illnesses and sent it off to the meeting's organizers in the United Kingdom. I received a response within a day. Not only did they invite me to Nairobi to speak, but I was also asked to moderate one of the panel discussions. Chairwoman Wangari Maathai was going to be very busy with the COP-5 proceedings, my invitation explained, and I would replace her on the panel. Wow, did I find a way in!

I flew to Nairobi. The session on traditional medicine was full of energy and excitement—as is often the case with a new conference topic that brings together like-minded people with extensive experiences from different parts of the globe. Discussions carried on into the late evenings, and plans were hatched to try to do something about the loss of indigenous healing knowledge in Africa. I gathered up the current theories, strategies, and challenges, and prepared myself to head back down to Tanzania to see what was going on in Maasailand.

I was a bit frightened, to be honest. I did not have the big, safe vehicles, badges, translators, and planned itineraries that my colleagues who worked for large development NGOs and aid agencies could rely on. What would the locals think of me? The night before I was scheduled to leave Nairobi on a four-hour bus ride south to Arusha, Tanzania, Wangari invited me to dinner at her home with a group of people also attending the COP-5. It was a wonderful evening. We told life stories, ate great food, and talked about being "change agents" in the world. As I was about to leave, I shared with Wangari my fear about my re-entry into Tanzania. She looked me straight in the eye and said "Tanya, you will be fine. The people you are going to find there will love you and take care of you. You *have* to go down there. Don't worry, you will know what to do." She gave me a big hug and sent me on my way.

Over the months since my return to Seattle from my first trip to Tanzania, I had kept in contact with some of the locals I had met. I had written to Sululu and his Maasai friends, telling them I was coming back and that I wanted to meet Maasai elders who could tell me more about their knowledge of healing and medicinal plants. They arranged to pick me up at the bus station in Arusha and help me work on my project proposal.

After some weeks of research and needs assessment in Tanzania, I headed back up to Nairobi to re-connect with Dr. Jessica Erdstieck, a colleague from Holland whom I had met at the conference and who was writing a book on spirit healing in Tanzania. We traveled together to Lake Naivasha to relax and to share some ideas about what we, as highly-educated Westerners, could actually do to conserve the traditional healing knowledge of indigenous Tanzanians. A project began to take shape.

On Christmas Eve, 2000, I received an email from the GEF regional director in Tanzania saying he was impressed with my proposal. He had some ideas for me about how to move ahead because he was already directing a large project focused on biodiversity conservation in East Africa. One of his project sites happened to be the location where I had proposed beginning research on the use of traditional medicine by the Maasai. We agreed to meet in Arusha and talk extensively soon after the beginning of the new year.

I was ready. I had declared my intention to do this work and live this life, and the pieces had fallen into place. I would be combining my years of education and research skills with my passion to discover the healing wisdom of the Maasai. The plan had been there for a long time. I simply needed quiet and focused attention to *see* the plan.

SUGGESTED PRACTICE

When you have moments of confusion or unhappiness in your daily life, take a moment to "rewind the video" and search for an underlying plot, rhythm to your life.

Which people, places and events pop out more strongly in hindsight? Is there a pattern?

Notice when statements, gestures, and actions truly spark you, engage you. Consider whether they may be signposts on your life's unfolding journey.

Practice paying attention, listening, and acting on your gut feelings more often. Take note of the results.

TALKING TO YOUR NATURE,
APPRECIATING ENGAI'S PLAN

A few months after my decade-long apprenticeship with the Maasai was complete and I had pursued further studies in indigenous Indian mind-body techniques and begun my own practice, I was asked to lead a group meditation at Gibb's Farm in Tanzania. Sululu was visiting the farm and asked if he could join with the visitors who were coming to the session. Afterward, I asked him what he thought of the practice. He said he particularly enjoyed the way in which I asked the participants to consider, "Who am I? What do I want?" and "How can I serve?" before they went into silence. He said it reminded him of what the Maasai do when they "talk to their nature."

I was curious to know more how my training in Vedic sciences—based on the Vedas, the ancient Hindu scripture—was similar to Maasai practices. Sululu reminded me that the Maasai belief in God, or *Engai*, is akin to what we term "Mother Nature." Deep down, our soul is connected to nature very directly. When there are a lot of changes happening in the community and an individual Maasai begins to feel overwhelmed, he or she will go off alone to "talk to their nature," sitting in silence under a tree and listening to what *Engai* is saying.

Sululu explained that sometimes you see elders sitting under an acacia tree with their eyes closed. You might think they are sleeping, but often times they are practicing what we tend to call "meditation." They sit cross-legged and close their eyes, asking, "*Engai narok*, you are everywhere on this earth. Where can I go without you? Where can I sit without you? You know me from when I was born, and now I start to open my mind."

"If there is anything bubbling up from the heart," Sululu explained, "you are open to talk to *Engai*, silently. You notice that the leaves are alive, the trees are alive, the water is alive, the wind is alive. I acknowledge that *Engai* put me here as one of the living so I say *ashe*, thank you for recommending me to be someone to control the nature. That means thanking *Engai* for putting you here as a human to do some things by harnessing and managing nature. You have to thank *Engai* for giving you air to breathe. You know, Maasai people feel very proud to be alive when they sit in this type of awareness."

I asked him how long he normally sits when he talks to his nature. He said it varied, from five or ten minutes up to an hour or more, depending on what was going on in his brain. "*Engai* knows what is in your heart before you talk," he added, "but just saying it makes it stronger."

"En" is the feminine gender prefix in the Maa language, and many vitally important nouns are feminine. *Engarre*, water. *Engop*, earth, world. *Engima*, fire. *Engijape*, air. We are all made up of a combination of the elements that exist in nature. When you talk to *Engai*, you know that *Engai* is the same as nature. The same water inside of you can also fall from the sky, as rain.

Maasais believe children are born with specific talents or gifts, whether for singing or dancing, counseling, healing with plants, healing spirits, or painting and plastering the walls of huts. When they recognize a gift, they support the person in expanding the gift. For example, Sululu explained, "when a person speaks diplomatically from an early age, people can see this. He is really good, he knows things. We then tell others to go speak to this person if they have a problem or we make him or her a chairperson."

While every Maasai has a godfather or godmother to help guide her in her life, some also have advisors. An *olage'lie* is a male advisor and an *enage'lie* is a female advisor. "It's important to keep secret who this person is," Sululu told me. "No one knows but you. And this person is different than the godfather. The *olage'lie* is for discussion, the godfather makes the last decision."

Some people have both godfather and godmother; some women like to receive advice from a man, some men like to talk with a woman. When young people know themselves well, they recognize what they can tell their parents, and what they can tell a trusted older man, woman, or friend. You begin to strike an equilibrium in what you say or show people, and what you don't. Open sharing is often filled with humor and light-heartedness, and the time of "talking with your nature" can be one of profound simplicity and honesty.

SUGGESTED PRACTICE

Where do you go to seek wisdom for yourself and for the important people in your life?

Take a moment to identify the advisor(s) in your life, both in the past and the present. Acknowledge and honor them and consider reconnecting if you have lost touch.

If you are in need of an *olage'lie* or *enage'lie,* reach out to the developing global network of wise elders and junior elders. Their wisdom can transform your life.

ACTING YOUR AGE SET

> "Soul is the meeting place of intelligence and wildness—healthy
> cultures and healthy individuals are those that strike the right
> balance between them. . . . There's a difference between nos-
> talgia and reappropriation. Nostalgia is the longing to return to
> the past, which is impossible. Re-appropriation is the retrieving
> from the past what we need in order to live fully human lives
> into the future. Growing up—as individuals and as a culture—
> involves in part the recognition that the traditions one rejected
> in adolescence, for whatever reason, preserved essential values
> for living life well. Re-appropriating those values doesn't mean
> living them naively or rigidly, but with the fully developed soul
> sense of an adult."
>
> —Jack Whelan, *Soul Food*

When I first asked Sululu to explain to me what the Maasai mean
when they talk about "age sets," he first described the group of
boys who are circumcised around the same time. Approximately
every fifteen years, the community's spiritual leader, the *laiboni*,
declares that it is time to create a new "age set." Over the next
seven or so years, waves of circumcisions are performed throughout Maasailand on boys between fourteen and twenty-two. This
marks their passage from boyhood into the warrior stage. It is a
rite of passage that encompasses preparation for the physical circumcision, the long healing and probationary period that follows,
and finally a special ceremony confirming warrior-hood.

Each boy is assigned a teacher, normally an uncle, who guides
him through the emotional, psychological, and physical aspects of

becoming a warrior. "The most important thing is we are taught the difference between how little boys behave and how men behave. I have an example," Sululu offered. "Little boys would sometimes eat while they are walking. Men sit down to eat. It is very serious. Also, warriors learn to defend the tribe and their property. They have responsibilities that boys don't have. When you become a warrior, and then later a junior elder and then an elder, you would never even think to behave like a little boy. In fact, you can easily see when people, especially those from other cultures that do not have these strong initiations, act like children. It can be funny to watch, although quite sad if the behavior is directed to one's parents or wife.

"I know many people around the world," he continued, "believe that cutting the penis, and certainly the clitoris of girls is awful. And it is, especially for girls. But with boys, I can tell you that you remember that pain forever. We do not use anesthesia but only a jump in cold river water first. We are not allowed to move or cry out during the procedure. It is powerful. There is no going back to childhood, physically or psychologically.

"I was at a circumcision ceremony for a family member the other day. We spent days talking and drinking honey beer and discussing current news from around Maasailand and the country. The morning of the cutting came. It is performed very early in the morning, when it is still dark. A traditional doctor skilled in using the knife performs the cutting. It was hard for me. I remembered the pain of my own circumcision, over thirty years ago, and tears came to my eyes. I couldn't cry then, but now tears just came."

It is interesting to me that these circumcisions happen in

waves, separated by a number of years, as a conscious way of creating what we call a "generation." Just as we have "Baby Boomers" and "Generation X," in Maasai culture the spiritual leader observes the current collection of younger boys and studies the group's common characteristics before he gives a name to their "age set." What is the group's personality type? Are they particularly outgoing, of service, or accomplished at tending cattle? The current Maasai age set coming into manhood in Tanzania is called *ilinyangulo*, which meets "boys who eat a lot." When they become junior elders in a few years, they will receive a new name.

I asked Sululu whether the fabric of a particular generation emanates from the biological level or the social level.

"Well, that's a good question! I never thought of that. I think it is a combination of the biological and social. A tendency may appear in a group of a particular age set, and then when it gets noticed and supported by the elders it starts to take on a self-fulfilling prophecy, I suppose you could say."

SUGGESTED PRACTICE

Think about a particular incident in the recent past in which you may have thought to yourself, "Why did I say that? That wasn't very mature of me." Is there a way for you to meet the person again and try again, this time apologizing and saying something wiser that better reflects your maturity?

Next time you have to make a big decision on something, ask for a bit of time. Write down all the thoughts that come to your mind. Note those that you would have acted on as a child, as an adolescent, and now.

Compare the several choices you might have made impulsively with the one you made after enough reflection. What is the difference?

BEING FEMALE

I was speaking with Sululu's niece, Zawadi, about the ritual in Maasai of giving cows to the family of a bride. And I was fascinated, because the concepts of gender and gender roles in Maasai culture, and in many traditional African cultures, have been the subject of great discussion and debate.

"When you say paying," she began, "well, you pay when you go to the shop, you pay the money and get the sugar, for example. But when it comes to a human being, maybe you still use that word 'paying' when you translate into English, but for me to be more comfortable with it I wouldn't translate it as 'paying cows to get a wife.' You can't even say exchange because you can't exchange cows and get a wife. Maybe if there is a better word to mark the exchange, then you come on this side. That is how I am looking at it. You have to understand that one side is losing something: a daughter, a sister, to go to the husband side. It is not about finding a replacement, you cannot replace a human being with cows. Think of it as giving cows to say, 'Thank you for giving us your daughter to take care of.' The cows are really a gift. If you try and use the word 'paying,' you will never really be able to 'pay' enough. I mean, the mother of the bride was pregnant for nine months, raised the child, then education is very expensive. The gift of cows is okay for me, it is kind, but it should not be translated as 'payment for a wife.' "

What I have been most fascinated by over the years is actually how both genders hold great power and respect in Maasai culture—not with the same underlying value systems in Western cultures, but male and females roles and their importance are honored nonetheless. The Maasai have great clarity about proper male and female roles and behaviors.

Zawadi continued her explanation of the marriage ritual: "I have thought about it for myself. If it is going to happen, I would like it to happen in the way I just explained to you. From my perspective though, I would prefer to see it as my family gaining a son as well, instead of me just going away. That is supposed to be the way it is in Maasai. But he is an in-law, not the same as the other sons."

While arranged marriages still occur in Maasailand, it is now common for young people to choose their spouse. Immediately, however, the families become involved. A girl will speak with her mother when a young man shows interest in her. If the mother does not know the man or knows he is from a troublesome family, then she will discourage her daughter. But she will encourage her daughter if she knows the possible husband comes from a good family. Daughters don't always take their mothers' advice, but they normally do, so by the time a girl brings her potential husband to her parents' home for a small ceremony of introduction, she should already be confident that they will approve of him.

I met Zawadi many years ago while she was still working on completing her education. She was determined to study law and achieve an advanced certificate—something very unusual for a Maasai woman who was born in a rural village. Sululu's brother, a medical doctor, had taken note of Zawadi's self-confidence and maturity when she was still a small child. He found a sponsor for her within his medical community who had taken her to boarding school in Kenya. By the time I met her, she was the most mature twenty-year-old I had ever met. She spoke Maa, Swahili, Kikuyu, French, and English, and could talk with me about profound and often complex issues and ideas.

Zawadi worked with our organization, Terrawatu, during one of our first projects in Maasailand. We took her and another young, educated Maasai woman to the Green Belt Movement headquarters in Nairobi to learn how Wangari Maathai had structured her tree-planting groups. Both women explained to me how in Maasai culture it would be very difficult to start any group with a leader who is not a man. I was concerned because I had hoped to replicate Wangari's practice of creating all-female groups, led by women. I took their advice, however—because they were Maasai themselves and because I respected their recommendations so highly. We created several groups in the villages of Mkonoo and Nadosoito, Tanzania that were mixtures of men and women or all women. Initially, all were led by men.

Because Zawadi was originally from one of the villages in the area where we were working, I asked her to speak to "her people" about deforestation, environmental destruction, and the importance of planting trees, both for firewood and for medicinal uses. Yet for months there was very little progress in the communities. When I asked her what she thought was going on she had a quick answer.

"Well, when I show up with you and Sululu in the villages, the community sees me one way, as having the power and respect afforded to me because I am connected with you, a white doctor, and Sululu, an elder. But they still know me as Zawadi, the little girl from the village. The girl who is supposed to marry, have children and help support a homestead with livestock and new farming techniques. All this talk about the environment, working for an NGO, and my own continued schooling to be a lawyer is confusing to them. For what benefit is that?"

Zawadi and I often shared long conversations about the role of women, not only in traditional African societies, but in the Western world as well. I explained to her that Americans are still figuring out gender roles as well—how does a woman have her own profession, raise a family and maintain a loving relationship and home all at the same time? I told her it wasn't easy.

She stuck to her plan to finish law school, despite the concerns of her village, and now practices as a lawyer in the south of Tanzania. She also teaches at a nearby law school. She is raising two children now, one of her own, and one she adopted from her sister, who passed away just after the birth of her fourth child. I asked how life is for her now.

"I remember years ago, when I went back to Nadosoito, some old women in the village said to me it is very good that I have gone so far in school and I have a job of my own. They said even though I may not get married, at least it would be good to have a child of my own. And those are the old women of the village! The same ones who said in the beginning it is not good for a woman to have a child without being married. I think they have seen the development and the way things are moving now. Even though my own decision is not based on them, deep down knowing their view now has given me comfort, in fact. I think a lot of things are changing, based on seeing specific people move through life."

Yet I can't help but wonder about Zawadi, and many other

modern Maasai women I know. Their womanhood shines; they have great pride and engender the deep respect of everyone who encounters them. I suspect that much of their strength and poise comes from being raised among such strong men.

She is deeply proud of her people, her culture. "I love being Maasai. Yes, there are some practices that are not good, like FGM (female genital mutilation), but it is the community I was brought up in. Maasais are not aggressive, unless they are provoked. I think that is human nature. I speak the language and I eat fish. Maasais traditionally don't eat fish. There is a graceful thing with Maasais. Even though I am living a very different life than my mother, I speak Maa to my children. It won't be easy because they don't have too many people to practice with, but it is important to me."

I knew that both Maasai men and women go through rigorous initiation ceremonies—rites of passage—as they move from childhood to adulthood. Male circumcision ceremonies and the events that lead up to them have been widely documented, but the female rituals were not well known to me or any outsiders. Those of us at Terrawatu had worked with some success to find alternatives to FGM in Maasai villages in Tanzania. I was now curious about the other aspects of how a girl becomes a woman in Maasai—the social and psychological elements of the initiation—and Zawadi suggested we talk about this with her mother.

I traveled to Nadosoito village with her to speak with her mother, Ndavukai, who greeted me very warmly. She asked the boys and men seated nearby to leave before we began our conversation. I promised her that some aspects of what she told me— those things she and other women considered secret—I would share only in private sessions with people I serve, in confidence.

Ndavukai began by explaining that "training is mainly done by your mother and a sister of your father. Also, the grandmother on the father's side, because in the boma a widowed mother lives with the husband's family. Training begins when a mother senses that her daughter has started her menstruation. She tells her sisters, and the sisters of the husband—the aunts of the daughter—to talk with the young woman. The mother does not do the training; she is too close to her daughter. Also, the child may not feel free to express herself with the mother. She usually feels more courage with the aunts."

In traditional times, there were two trainings—the first at puberty and the second prior to circumcision. Because the practice of female circumcision is finally coming to an end, the women are finding ways to shift their focus to teaching the woman how to live with a husband, how not to have affairs. The Maasai now acknowledge that girls grow faster than men, biologically. Most Maasai girls begin their first menstrual cycle around fourteen or fifteen, which marks an important movement into adulthood. Girls are instructed to stop playing and to begin to behave like a woman. They are also warned to be very careful with men because they are not to get pregnant.

I asked Ndavukai what Maasai women do to attract men. "They wear special clothes, beads, and they dance. Men are told not to have sexual relations with women until they are circumcised. So men cannot touch women until then."

She described some of the plants that are used specifically to treat menstrual cramps, infertility, and to ease pain during pregnancy. All of the plant medicines are consumed in ritualistic ways, and both the professional healer and the female patient perform the rituals with deep intention and attention. Maasai women perceive preparing for childbirth as a group effort. They support each other to make sure it all works out in the best way possible.

A pregnant woman is given herbs and roots from certain trees that are meant to clean her stomach, purify her blood system, and keep her healthy. At the birth of a baby, a midwife usually attends, helping to cut the umbilical cord as she announces to the newborn, "You are now responsible for your life in as much as I am responsible for mine." *Ing'urai keon maing'urai keon.* Ashe Engai. Literally, "Hold your heart while I hold mine. Thank God."

When a child is born it is first given a "pet name," an *embolet*, meaning "opener." Sometimes the name is in reference to a cute identifying mark on the infant's body, her smile, or her temperament as she enters the world. The child continues to be known by this name until given a proper name, often not for many years. When a growing child begins to exhibit the personality traits of a family member who has passed away, it is believed the spirit of that person may have been reborn in the new person, a process the Maasai call "spiritual genetics," and the child is often formally given the dead person's name.

BEING MALE

During the process of preparing for circumcision, a Maasai boy is taught what is important in becoming a man. Long ago, this meant getting married, having children, then perhaps taking one or more additional wives, and raising cattle. Even today, men gain respect in the community in these ways. Accumulating wisdom is a very strong motivating goal in Maasai culture—wise elders are deeply revered—and men seek wisdom with much the same dedication that they build their cattle herds.

I was surprised when I first discovered that grown Maasai men are not ashamed to cry. In fact, when overcome with grief, I have seen many Maasai men shake with emotion. They really feel it. When I first met Sululu in Tanzania, he was leading a tourist group to Tarangire National Park for a wildlife safari. I sat in the passenger seat of a Land Cruiser and tried to make small talk with him as we drove, but I noticed that he seemed sad.

When I asked if he was okay, he said, "I am thinking about my neighbor. He died last night in a motorcycle accident. Today I will be sad. I need to grieve this." And he did. The following day, however, he was exuberant, talkative, and happy, entertaining our group with stories of his own circumcision and the time he killed a lion and brought the tail to his father, so his father would be proud.

I was amazed. This strong and powerful man who had killed a lion with nothing more than a pointed stick and a spear could also be quiet and emotionally sensitive, and he could modulate his emotions as he chose. It was as if he had perfected the art of yin and yang balancing. As I met more and more members of the Maasai tribe, both men and women, almost all of them were capable of this same emotional dance. I learned that their culture provides clear scripts for the performances they necessarily play out in their lives. When the heart feels something, you express it. Over-thinking things is an attempt to dampen the feeling and is not healthy. During the lessons boys are given about becoming an adult, they are taught to free their emotions, and to feel and speak the truth, limiting stress. Girls are taught this as well, and both genders learn how to dance with the opposite sex in a kind of emotional play.

When a young boy is preparing to become a warrior, a "godfather" is chosen by his parents. According to Sululu, "it has to be someone who knows enough about the family but is not too emotionally attached. For example, a father cannot be the godfather to his son." A vital aspect of becoming an adult is learning how to live with wildlife, which includes lions, elephants and leopards. "Animals are aggressive; you learn not to disturb them. If you love them, they will love you. *Engai* put the animals together with us. Animals can teach us things. You learn how to live together on this earth; everyone has a place and has a right to live here."

In recent times, as the balance between land, wildlife, population, and economics has shifted, a few Maasai have chosen to kill wildlife that have taken their livestock. Traditionally, this was rare, because the Maasai believe that *Engai* created all animals—cows and wildlife as well—and that each animal has to be true to its nature. Because of the increasing imbalances in the ecosystems, the role of warriors in protecting both tribe and livestock has become more complex as wildlife increasingly prey on the docile cows and sheep.

SUGGESTED PRACTICE

If you are a woman, think about your essential female-ness. What makes you a woman? Spend a part of each day by yourself, honoring these elements, and, when possible, with other women. When you are with important men in your life, evoke those feminine aspects with respect and pride.

If you are a man, think about your essential male-ness. What makes you a man? Spend a part of each day by yourself honoring these elements, and when possible, with other men. When you are with important women in your life, evoke these male aspects with respect and pride.

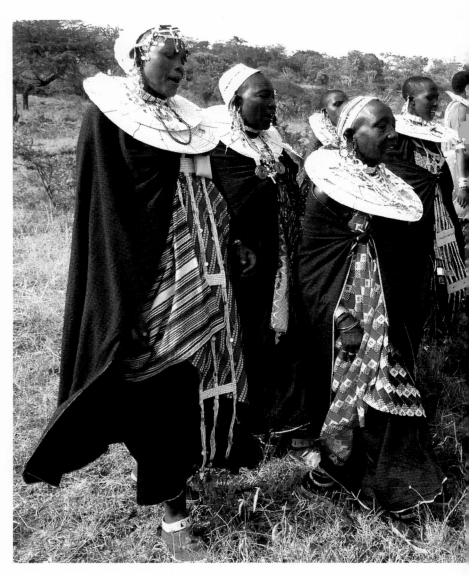

Maasai women celebrating the coming of age of male warriors in Monduli, Tanzania

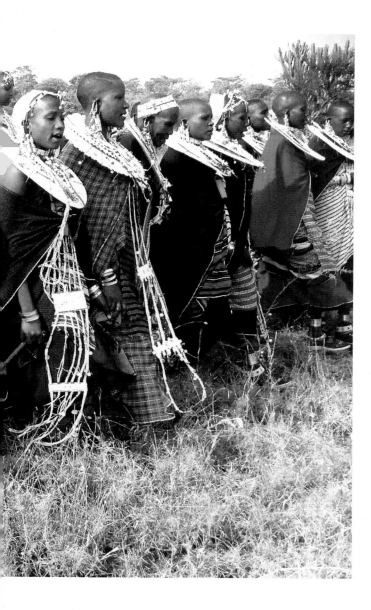

LEARNING YOUR WEAKNESSES

During one of our conversations, Sululu mentioned that at some point every young warrior would be asked by his godfather or an uncle, "What is your particular weakness?" I didn't understand, so he spoke more frankly. "You know, everybody has something he has a weakness towards, either tobacco, alcohol, sex, or stealing." I recognized he was talking about what we tend to call addictions and was fascinated to hear how an ancient culture understood what I assumed to be a modern problem.

Sululu explained that the Maasai believe everyone is born with a propensity to crave a particular external stimulus so much that it becomes an unhealthy part of one's life. This weakness, he said, usually first appears when warriors begin living independently from their parents and are free from prohibitions imposed by them. Before a warrior can be initiated into junior elder status, he must search deep in his soul and reveal to his godfather the specific thing he knows will be a weakness throughout his life.

When a warrior is first asked about his weakness, he is cautioned not to answer right away. Instead, he is encouraged to go off alone for a length of time and "talk to his nature." Only after he has reflected at length on his past behavior with alcohol or snuff or his sexual behaviors does he then return to his godfather and admit his weakness. Once it is identified, he begins to manage this addictive element of his personality with the godfather's support and wisdom. As circumstances change in life, what a warrior is addicted to may change. If it does, the godfather remains ready to encourage a similar process again.

"Everybody is addicted to something," Sululu maintained. "In Maasailand we ask you as a young person to think deeply about what your weakness is. The place inside you that feels insatiable, where you keep coming back to try and fulfill. Yet it never is satisfied. For some people the craving is nicotine, and they keep feeding it with tobacco, or, as you people use, cigarettes. For others it is alcohol. For some it is sex or stealing property or energy from other people. Sometimes we don't even notice our addictive behavior, but sometimes we do. A strong addiction is some behavior we are fully aware of causing us to deviate from living a productive life, yet we do it anyway. We say we can't help it."

It seems to me the Maasai approach addiction in a very healthy way. They simply ask everyone point-blank to what he is addicted, believing that if you admit to your own weaknesses early on, you have a much better chance of managing them. You can leave the job that is causing you stress and you can leave the group of friends or companions who encourage your addiction. By proclaiming to your close community what your weakness is, its members can help you manage it, too.

I asked Sululu if you can also be addicted to good things in Maasai, and he agreed this was possible. A person can be *arip*, for example; someone who keeps giving advice, helps people constantly, never provokes. Yet the danger is he or she can give too much and lose the necessary balance between caring for others and caring for oneself.

You cannot care for others if you are not strong and healthy. When people become addicted to helping others and ignore their own health in the process, it's important for others to remind them to take care, because otherwise the whole community will suffer. Everybody needs to stay strong and healthy, regardless of their purpose in life. Addictions often form precisely around the place that is potentially strongest in the person, appearing as the shadow side of a light-giving gift. The Maasai take this very seriously, as should we.

SUGGESTED PRACTICE

Check in with yourself. What would you say is your biggest weakness or addiction, one that perhaps you have had since childhood? Is it towards alcohol, tobacco, sex, food, sugar? You may crave it because it feels like it would alleviate subtle pain or suffering, but after you indulge in it, the pain is still there.

Next time you have a hankering for X, stop yourself and ask why? Is there something else you can do instead? Some other, healthier, behavior?

It may not be easy to see what your weakness is. Put yourself in a situation where you are naked to your truth. Tell your "godfather" or closest mentor, someone you respect highly.

THE FAMILY MEETING

Fundamental to knowing who you are in Maasai culture is understanding your interactions within your extended family. Magically
healthy and happy families do not exist in Maasai culture any
more than they do in modern western societies. Conflicts and suffering arise in Maasai families just as they do all over the world.
What became apparent to me, however, was the fascinating way in
which issues are addressed and problems worked through in the
Maasai families I have had the privilege to get to know.

In the Maasai world, the health and happiness of any individual family member is inextricably linked to the health and
happiness of the whole family. It is truly impossible to ignore the
wellbeing of a family member. If you try, your own wellbeing will
eventually begin to deteriorate.

When I first arrived in Africa, I had some knowledge of the importance of family members who have died, and the huge amounts
of time and effort people in traditional cultures spend on family
matters. In fact, I was curious to learn the truth about "ancestor
worship," which as far as I knew, may have been related to some
people's ability to actually interact with the spirits of the dead. The
Maasai helped me understand that honoring and continuing to engage with your entire extended family—including those who are deceased—is not a spooky activity at all. We all should really be more
aware of this realm of understanding; in fact, it can shed great light
on our own present-day thoughts and behaviors.

I like to refer to African ancestor awareness as "primordial
genetics." The physical genes of our ancestors literally live within

us, of course. The behaviors that are coded by these genes form the foundation of who we are—our wants, needs and actions. Each one of us is the sum of the genes of our ancestors, passed on from generation to generation.

Throughout history, parents and children, brothers and sisters grow as branches of our family tree, and we display our foliage in unique yet quite predictable ways. Yet no one pays too much attention until the wind blows and branches get tangled, or a branch breaks off and dies. Then family conflict—and sometimes crisis—emerge.

In Maasai culture, family meetings are called only when circumstances beg for one. When a series of unexplained illnesses or accidents plague a family, for example, a meeting is called to discuss what may be disturbing the roots of the family tree. Or, at those times when there is unrest and problems arise in relationships within the family fabric itself, it is time to gather together, take a step back from daily activities and look at and discuss the bigger picture.

Who is not pulling his or her weight? Who is disrespecting his or her power? This process of investigation and reflection involves both people who are alive and those who have passed on. The spirits of family members who have died remain vital parts of the family. Those who are still living need to take the time now and then to "talk to their nature" and tap into the plan *Engai* has laid out.

Maasai families tend to be quite large—especially when a male head of household has multiple wives who have given birth to numerous children. It is not unusual for someone to have *dozens* of brothers, sisters, aunts, uncles, and cousins. Yet like many

African tribes, the Maasai do not use the terms that are the equivalent of "aunt," uncle," or "cousin." Any sister of your mother or father is your "little mother," and any brother of your father or mother is your "little father." Every son or daughter of your "little father" or "little mother" is your brother or sister.

Not everyone in this entire extended family is required to attend a family meeting when one is called. As long as there is representation from the side or sides of the family that are directly involved in whatever issue is at stake, there is a "quorum," so to speak, and a meeting, led by the family chairperson, can proceed.

Family meetings are not easy, anywhere, yet in traditional Maasailand, family meetings are an important way to heal both individual and whole families. Healing is a social activity for the Maasai—a time to open your heart, speak the truth and share love and support with those who matter most to you. Current conflicts almost always have long histories that bear revisiting from time to time, because the past often provides insight into whatever is plaguing the present.

When a family meeting is called, Maasais often have to make real sacrifices to attend. Travel is not easy and is often expensive, and taking time away from one's daily activities can be a burden to others as well. Yet sacrifice is precisely what ignites the intention and attention that are necessary for people to participate fully in a meeting aimed at healing and transformation.

The location of the meeting is important, too. A distinct type of energy emerges from meetings that are held within closed doors compared with those that are held outside. As you travel around Maasailand, you can often see a circle of people dressed in traditional clothing, sitting under a tree, talking—a sign that a meeting is taking place. Talking outside, in nature, is preferred because outside the confines of walls and buildings, the intensity of discussion is easily dissipated into the natural environment. This is also part of the healing and transformation. Heated arguments can cool down quickly when emotions are released into air and space.

"After the blessing, the first thing we do when we have a meeting—it doesn't matter whether it is morning, afternoon or

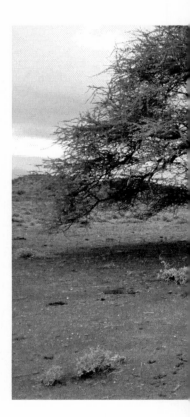

Maasai meeting under an acacia tree

evening—is we have to ask each other "How are you?" Sululu explained. "We go around the circle and everyone gets a chance to talk. One person can take even five minutes. *Aribioto? . . . aya . . . mmm.* We tell each other about health. 'I am fine, we are fine, the kids, we suffer from no water,' or 'the rain is good.' Many things to tell each other so everyone understands what is going on." No one's experience exists in a vacuum, and this initial check-in time helps everyone begin to start to see the bigger picture.

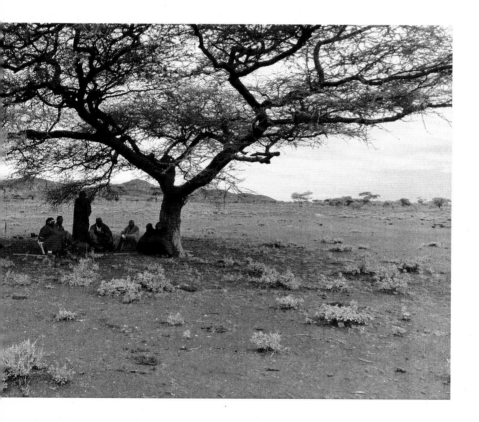

"After we finish, we can say okay, everyone is happy, everyone is doing great, then we can begin the talking about the meeting."

"What if someone is not doing well?" I asked.

"Well, then we try to help, maybe someone is sick and someone knows someone who can help with healing. Or, if someone knows where there is water to bring cows that need water. Or, say they are sorry to hear someone has died. You have to give encouragement for the situation. You can't go through, directly. First, you notice when someone is not happy. Try to make them comfortable and then gently find out the news. The way you approach people and ask them how they are is the way we bring people together, to make symbols of peace and love."

I have integrated this Maasai practice of beginning meetings by having people "check in" with each other for years. What is amazing every time is that as each person talks, themes emerge among the group. People are either struggling with family relationships, or have issues with their bosses, almost as if the trouble is "in the air." Once we begin to recognize that our problems are not unique to us, we feel connected to each other in a deeper way, and at that point it's easy to carry on with the business at hand without being strangers.

Sululu explained that Maasai family meetings always have a chairperson, but everyone in attendance is expected, even required to talk. "We don't really have 'chiefs' in Maasailand, they are not really accepted. But we do have leaders. Each family has a leader, and then each village has a leader." A chief counselor is called a *olaiguenani*. "People sit in a circle. When someone is ready to speak, he or she stands and takes hold of a talking stick.

Tajarra oljani. 'Make wide a tree.' When more people come in, they are welcomed. There is no alcohol involved, only when the meeting is finished. We never eat and talk. The attention is all on the matter of discussion. We wait until the meeting is finished before eating. Then we celebrate because we have resolved something. It is a good feeling."

The family meeting is a sacred event, a time to get everything out in a shared and intentional way. Gossiping or leaking secrets to only a few without proper attention, respect, and follow-up can make matters worse—and from my experience, the Maasai can be very open yet secretive at the same time. They play and joke and appear not to have a care in the world, yet inside a family meeting the seriousness of the emotions, accusations, and the ways in which people speak to each other can become intense. Issues can take hours, days, or months to resolve, but when they do, light-heartedness and collective peace inevitably return. The contrasts can be stark.

In our own modern lives, our "families" often extend to include close friends and even colleagues. As we spend more and more time with people other than our own blood relations and forge partnerships involving money and property, the word "family" has come to mean your people, your tribe. And problems can arise in these larger families in exactly the same way they do among people who are true kin. Ultimately, to truly know yourself is to know your position within a family consciousness—and to hold this position with pride, respect, flexibility and love. It's vital in every context to engage in opportunities for resolving conflict, because those resolutions always bring positive growth and transformation.

SUGGESTED PRACTICE

When trying to resolve a problem with a friend, family member, or co-worker, take a moment to consider all the people who are related to that problem, even tangentially. Consider inviting everyone involved to a meeting at which you seek resolution.

Consider where to bring people together, whether inside a house or outside in nature. Plan the location carefully.

Sit in a circle, elect a chairman or chairwoman whose job it is to keep everyone on "power point."

Open the meeting with a blessing to appeal to a higher force to guide the group towards a healthy resolution of the issue at hand.

Before beginning the discussion, go around the circle and ask each person to take five minutes or so to describe how she is and what is focal in her life at the moment.

Create a literal "talking stick" out of an object close at hand, to help everyone stay focused on the person speaking, offering her undivided attention with no interruptions. This also encourages the person speaking to say something that is worthy of the listeners' valuable time.

Do not serve food or alcohol until after a resolution has been reached. Refreshments can be distracting and encourage people to fall asleep or lose focus.

Take time to celebrate at the meeting's conclusion. Then, take time to rest.

4.

Plant Medicine

Terrawatu, the name of the organization I co-founded with Sululu in 2000, was initiated in Tanzania with a grant from the United Nations Development Program (UNDP). The name came to me in a dream. *Terra* means "earth" in Latin (and in my beloved Italian!) and *watu* is Swahili for "people." People of the Earth. Sululu and I agreed that the best way to achieve our parallel goals of creating vital development projects and providing Westerners with learning about the traditional healing wisdom of the Maasai was to create an officially recognized non-governmental organization (NGO), which would facilitate the attraction of both financial support and volunteers who would be eager to come and assist.

The UNDP grant to Terrawatu was for the study and documentation of the use of traditional plant medicine in Maasai communities in a district called Monduli, in northern Tanzania. This activity was part of a larger biodiversity project that was examining the conservation status of flora and fauna in three cross-border sites in

Kenya, Tanzania, and Uganda. We created a team composed of both English- and Maa-speaking members, many of whom were from the Monduli area. We gathered information by going out with both elders and children on "plant walks," and having long conversations over tea inside Maasai homes. I was delighted by how many children would sing the names and uses of numerous plants for me, especially in the remote areas. It was a part of their upbringing, part of learning how to survive in the bush.

As I sat on the slope of a hill overlooking savannah lands and Lake Manyara surrounded by a group of Maasai elders one afternoon, Sululu carefully translated the incredibly complex information people were sharing with me about specific plants and their uses for treating everything from malaria to the opportunistic infections caused by HIV/AIDS. I, in turn, diligently wrote down everything Sululu said. During a break in the conversation, one of the elders wanted to know, "Why are you writing everything down? Why can't you just put it in your head like we have?" I was struck by how differently he and I had been trained to learn.

This was my first introduction to the vast array of plants used medicinally in Maasai culture; the final report my colleagues and I wrote would eventually include tables listing *hundreds* of plants, their Maasai names, associated Latin scientific names; their traditional uses, and their current "conservation status"—meaning whether the plants were still widely available or were in danger of becoming extinct.

As our project unfolded, we discovered, to our dismay, that in relatively urbanized areas—which over the years had received more impact from the outside world than the rural areas where we worked—people tended to be embarrassed or even ashamed to speak with us about traditional medicine. Outsiders evidently had persuaded them that the use of plant medicine was primitive, and even dangerous. Understandably, many Western visitors to Africa have real concerns about the "witchdoctors" and assorted snake-oil peddlers who operate without any moral code and who have given traditional African medicine a bad name. Many missionaries and development workers have encouraged the Maasai to stop using their traditional medicine and seek health-care only at newly constructed conventional medicine clinics. While this was a positive development in theory, few of these new clinics could be staffed with properly trained doctors, let alone with a reliable supply of allopathic medicines.

People were gradually losing their traditional medicine and healing knowledge and, at the same time, failing to be well-served by modern health science. My team took this as a call to action. I felt strongly that the debate about the relative value of Western medicine versus traditional medicine was *not* something on which we wanted to spend our time. It was clear: people were getting more and more *un-well*, both in developed and underdeveloped communities. The opportunity to unearth and nurture rapidly disappearing indigenous medicine knowledge from Africa and discover its parallels to cutting-edge mind-body medicine from the West seemed to be a bridge very worth building.

First, however, we needed to keep this traditional knowledge from disappearing. I knew that simply keeping names of plants and their uses tucked in a large binder in a development office was not going to do much to keep the knowledge alive. The work had to include the rich and open discussions among the Maasai we had just conducted for the UN project. Sululu and his apprentices needed to be more than translators of words. They would have to find a way to speak with their people at the level of their cultural consciousness.

Time was short. We pressed on as rapidly as we could to both unearth ancient wisdom and re-kindle dignity and pride in Maasai communities for the precious resource their ancestors had handed down to them. We were an unlikely team—an American Ph.D. sociologist inspired by modern technologies and a Maasai elder-healer and naturalist who was passionate about the old ways of his people.

For four years we traveled to dozens of Maasai villages speaking with people we encountered about the usefulness of traditional medicine and traditional cultural practices that were healthy for communities. When we encountered old cultural practices that did not seem healthy anymore—or, like female circumcision, which were *never* healthy—we explored ways to replace them. I would bring news and ideas from my journeys to America, Europe, and India, and collectively we laid plans for marrying the good of the old with the good of the new.

We discovered from our original work in Monduli that some trees were being over-harvested for commercial purposes, or incorrectly harvested by people without proper training, causing the trees to die. This prompted Terrawatu to establish nurseries to cultivate both trees and medicinal plants, following the grassroots model developed by Wangari Maathai's Greenbelt Movement in Kenya. We chose plants that were most commonly used by the

Maasai to help motivate them to care for the nurseries, which was always a challenge in the most drought-prone areas. Sululu and Zawadi explained to their people that it was important to conserve traditional medicinal plant species and to re-learn the uses of a number of plants which nowadays were being overlooked.

Many Maasai recently had become convinced that Western medicine was superior to their traditional plant medicine, and so no longer sought out or shared the knowledge of what plants could be used to cure specific illnesses. Conserving indigenous knowledge is never simple in these contemporary times. It is difficult to explain to people that "new" may not always be better. It can be even more challenging to describe how highly-educated scientists now are finding evidence for time-tested truths about human health that people like the Maasai have always known.

NATURE HEALING—EMBUKUNOTO ENGLISHUUNOTO

Meeta enemeidima pookin ake Enemeidima
atunjani otwa meshukunyei.
Every disease has a cure except death.

Curiously, the Maasai use the same word for both "plant" and "medicine" —*ilkeek* in the singular and *olchani*, plural. They believe all plants are medicine, although there are many for which we have not yet discovered their medicinal use. Many of the medicines we have in modern pharmacies today were originally derived from plants. For example, aspirin (*acetyl salicylic acid*) comes from the bark of the white willow tree; compounds extracted from the Pacific yew tree (*Taxus brevifolia*) led to the identification of the chemical taxol, which is used to treat ovarian cancer, and the chemotherapy drug oncovin was derived from the Madagascan periwinkle (*Catharanthus roseus*).

We discovered during our original UNDP research that about fifty percent of the plant medicines the Maasai described were used to prevent disease and about half were used to cure illness. Over centuries, their knowledge of efficacious plants developed only through experience, trial and error, and sharing from person to person across generations—the knowledge often kept alive in the lyrics of songs. Most Maasai living in rural villages know the most commonly used medicinal plants and how to prepare them, but a few people—who make the subject their specialty—become healers. "Some had more illness in their extended family and needed to learn a lot and learn fast," Sululu said. "People in the village then start to know who knows more and go to them as experts. Becoming a professional herbalist is a calling."

THE FIVE MOST COMMONLY USED PLANTS BY THE MAASAI FOR MEDICINAL PURPOSES

1) *Ilodua (Embelia schimperi)* is found in the highland areas. Crushed dried fruits of this tree are popular mixed in black tea to help maintain general health and ward off colds. It is most commonly used by the Maasai as a purgative for cleansing the stomach and as an anthelmintic (kills worms). *Ilodua* has many benefits and there is solid scientific evidence to support its antioxidant and anti-inflammatory effects.

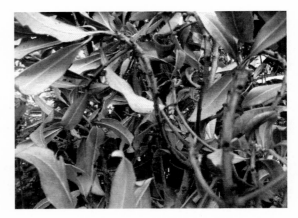

1) Leaves of the Ilodua plant

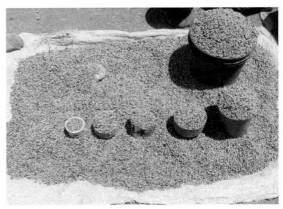

Dried berries from the Ilodua plant for sale at a local traditional medicine market

2) Oloisuki (Zanthoxylum chalybeum) grows ubiquitously in the forest and cool, shady mountain areas throughout Maasailand. One of the most popular Maasai medicines, often taken twice or more times daily as a tea made from its dried stem bark and/or crushed dried fruits. It helps prevent disease and maintain a general state of good health and well-being. At higher doses, *oloisuki* is used to treat many diseases from malaria to erectile dysfunction.

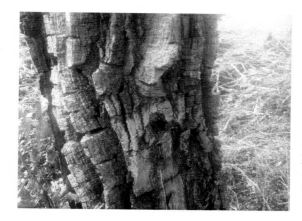

2) Bark of the Oloisuki plant after a piece has been harvested for medicine

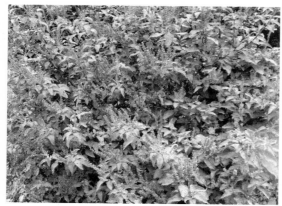

3) Field of Elemurran plants

3) Elemurran (Ocimum suave) is a member of the mint family found in the open in the highland areas, quite commonly on the edges of grasslands in "hedges" and among other shrubs. These plants need exposure to sunlight to grow well; when they get it, they produce an aromatic oil. The dried leaves and stems of *elemurran* are used to treat upper respiratory problems such as cough, flu, and general colds, as well as eye and ear issues and

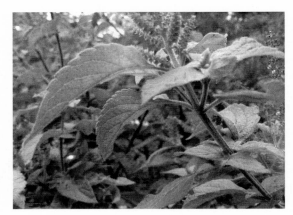

Close-up view of the leaves of the Elemurran plant

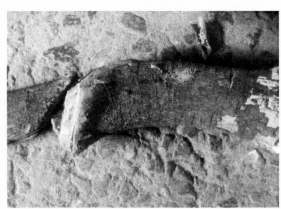

4) Dried stem bark of the Orkokola plant

general pain. It also helps lower blood cholesterol. Similar to the plant *Ocimum tenuiflorium*, holy basil, used in Indian Ayurvedic medicine as a tonic for a variety of ailments.

4) Orkokola (Rhamnus staddo) is a shrub native to East Africa that grows throughout Maasailand. This medicine, made from either dried stem bark or root bark, shares similar active chemical con-

116

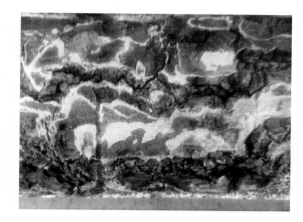

5) Bark of the Osokonoi plant

stituents with *aloe vera*. It is used topically to relieve pain, maintain healthy liver, pancreas, and kidney function, as well as having anti-cancer properties. During the forest retreat, known as *orlpul*, *orkokola* is used together with other related plant species as a tonic to cleanse the blood and restore health.

5) *Osokonoi (Warburgia salutaris/ugandensis)* is commonly known as the "pepper-bark tree." This large tree is found throughout eastern and southern Africa, and is considered to be a "hot" medicine that has the power to cure severe diseases. The dried stem bark of *osokonoi* contains different bioflavonoids, which are present in so-called "superfoods," and potent antibiotic compounds that help reduce pain and inflammation and fight tumor growth. *Osokonoi* also contains one of the same active ingredients as in *oloisuki*, which helps alleviate erectile dysfunction.

Virtually all of the hundreds of plants traditionally used by the Maasai to prevent and cure minor and major diseases contain multiple active ingredients that act synergistically. Most modern allopathic medicines, in contrast, have one known chemical with one directed pharmacological effect. Because plant medicines so often have multiple active ingredients, dispensing them becomes something of an art form. Understanding the combination of therapeutic actions in specific plants and how they can be used by individual patients seeking to prevent or cure diseases is a highly developed skill that includes a significant dose of intuition.

When people ask me if plant medicine really works, I tend to remind them that over two thousand years of successful use and extensive empirical evidence both support its efficacy, not only in Maasailand but throughout Africa and among cultures that have relied on nature's pharmacy for millennia. Central to the ways in which plant-based medicines prevent, lessen, and even cure illness is the connection between our physical bodies and our environment, the ritual use of medicinal plants, and one's close community.

According to the Maasai, illness can originate either from the outside environment or from inside the body. The Maasai believe problems inside the body develop from an imbalance of nutrients. And much illness is the result of an individual body being out of balance with its environment. The Maasai prepare and use their medicines to maintain the body, treat its diseases, rehabilitate it, and even improve the constitution of a healthy person. "Keeping yourself strong is the best way to handle a disease or illness when it shows up," Sululu maintained. "To be strong means a person has a lot of energy, a body in good shape, a good state of health, being able to eat a lot, and first of all, to be able to carry out one's duties."

After spending lots of time in Nadosoito, Sululu's niece Zawadi's home village, people began to tell us there was less illness years ago when there were more trees. A place with lots of trees means the air is cleaner, they explained. Trees contribute to keeping the residents who live among them stronger and healthier than people who live in deforested areas. Elders believed when someone moves to a new climate, or experiences the change of seasons, the body attempts to adapt. Yet in the process of adapting to new conditions, the body sometimes becomes sick in response to this change. Health is recovered by bringing the bodily elements back in balance with natural circumstances, because all events and states of being are linked with nature.

Like many indigenous cultures, the Maasai envision disease as a projection on the body of social and cosmic disorder. Therefore, when the Maasai treat a sick person, whether he is suffering from a mild ailment or a serious disease, they employ natural substances to restore order and reaffirm the boundary that separates life from death. It is a holistic approach in which the body is seen as a part of a larger system that is intimately interconnected with nature.

The natural environment can be described in many ways in the Maa language. Low-lying savanna pastures that are generally dry and hot with very few permanent water sources generally are known as *olpurkel* landscapes, which support short, nutrient-rich grasses that are high in salinity. An *osupuko* landscape is mountain pasture land, colder and wetter, with tall, nutrient-poor grasses that are low in salinity and mineral content. Livestock and wild animals utilize *olpurkel*, or "hot" zones, in the rainy season when the rich short grasses are abundant. During the dry season—

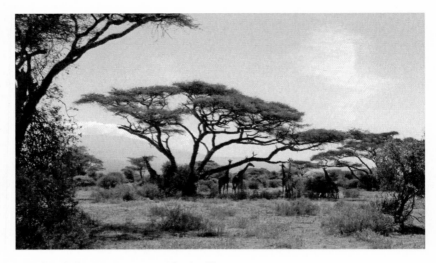

An olpurkel environment (with giraffe)

when the grass in the hot zone is reduced to stubble—the animals
are moved to the colder and higher *osupuko* regions. *Olpurkel* and
osupuko are relative, of course, and are dependent on climate and
climate changes. The transition zones between them are mixes
of both. Yet the distinction between the two terms, the two landscapes, is central to the Maasai concept of "hot" and "cold," not
only in relation to landscapes but to other aspects of the environment, including plants that are transformed into medicines.

   A tree is either hot, *oirowua*, or cold, *airobi*. "Hot" trees do
not give much shade and often have thorns. A "cold" tree offers
shade and protection. Cold trees are employed to create objects
in Maasai rituals, because no one wishes for "hot" results. Maasai
health care incorporates both a homeopathic approach—in which
like treats like—and the notion of harmonizing body-mind imbal-

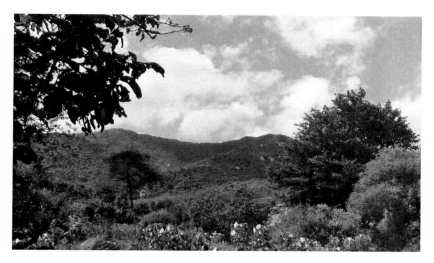

An osupuko landscape

ances. "Hot" medicines are used with great care; they are bitter and potent and tend to be used only to treat complicated diseases. "Cold" medicines, on the other hand, are more palatable and are often made into soups to maintain general good health.

"A skilled healer will speak with a patient for a long time to understand the root of the problem and decide which type of remedy will be most effective," Sululu told me. "There are also phases of energy, the energy patterns one's body goes through. A time to create, a time to incubate, a time to rest. Knowing how to sense the difference is a gift. Knowing what fuel works at what time is a special understanding. In old times, Maasai healers only took payment, cows or food, *after* a patient was healed. The idea is to allow the doctor to do his work, with the focus on healing the patient, instead of making a lot of money."

SOUP FOR A SISTER

> I believe that the difference between the indigenous world and
> the industrial world has mostly to do with speed—not about
> whether one world needs to have ritual and the other doesn't....
> Speed is a way to prevent ourselves from having to deal with
> something we do not want to face. So we run from these symp-
> toms and their sources that are not nice to look at. To be able
> to face our fears, we must remember how to perform ritual. To
> remember how to perform ritual, we must slow down.
> —Malidoma Patrice Some, *Ritual*

Those of us living in modern societies have come to expect
medicines and health treatments to work very rapidly. Fast-paced
lifestyles present an important challenge to the holistic practice
of traditional medicines. Traditional Maasai medicine, and most
traditional medicine systems, is most successful when patient and
healer have access to a large pharmacopeia of medicinal plants
used for both prevention and cure of disease, the active concern
and support of an extended family, and *time*.

The Maasai who still live primarily in the bush maintain an
intimate connection between the natural world and their own
bodies. There is a permeable boundary between their own skin
and the space around them. It is as if the flow of whatever is going on outside, from sunshine to rain, cold weather to hot, finds
its way inside the body. They will tell you that nature's rhythms
move slowly in relation to modern clocks.

In the Western world, a by-product of extraordinary modern

advancements in medicine and technological procedures that treat the body has been a disintegration of the once-intimate bond between the mind, heart, and emotions and the natural environment. "Fixing" the body has outpaced a necessarily parallel focus on re-balancing every aspect of an individual, something indigenous societies still understand very well.

I remember getting a call when I was back in Seattle for a period of weeks from a friend who hoped I had some painkillers, because she had thrown out her back. Her question surprised me because, like me, she was a practicing yogi and more likely to use gentle asanas to relieve back pain than to pop pills. I knew she must be in serious pain. I told her I had nothing in the house but that I could stop by a drugstore and bring something to her, mentioning, too, that Sululu was visiting from Tanzania. I explained to him that she was really sick and we needed to go bring her medicine.

"You are going to cook for her, right? It is dinner time; she has to eat," he said. I was already back in the mind-set of Seattle culture, I quickly realized. In Tanzania, of course, not only would I go to a sister's home to help her get better, I would stay with her. Women did it for me in Tanzania—as did the friend who had come to my home in Tanzania to make me *mtori*, banana soup, when I was sick with malaria. She stayed with me all day, cooking and talking and simply being with me.

So, I was preparing a bag with vegetables and soup bouillon when the phone rang. It was my friend, saying she had found some painkillers. When I told her I was coming anyway and was going to cook dinner for her, she said, "Oh, don't do that, I can order take-out online and have it delivered."

I thought, yes, of course she can. This is Seattle, where you don't have to leave your computer screen and everything can be delivered to your doorstep. But I also experienced a sadness. I know a big part of healing involves having your people close to you help you. So many times in Maasailand I have watched a sick person receive a plant remedy in the setting of a secure and comfortable room, surrounded by her close people. Yes, the chemical compounds in the plant medicine acted on her illness, but the presence, singing, thoughts, and good wishes of her friends were also vital to her return to good health.

The "modern" way of attending to illness typically involves the mechanical exchange of medicine and advice for money during short and quick sessions with doctors, or pharmacists, or even alternative healers. And many people, of course, attempt to keep their illnesses secret. The ancient idea that we are all on earth to help heal each other has become lost in the sea of contemporary self-sufficiency. I doubt this is true progress.

SUGGESTED PRACTICE

Next time a friend or family member is sick, stop what you are doing and pay attention.

Consider going to visit and make soup or other food for your patient.

Make a recipe based on your own cultural tradition or the tradition of your patient—comfort food, in other words, food that's familiar and savory.

Spend time just talking, allowing your patient to share freely.

TALKING TO PLANTS

As we began our work, I had been asked by my UNDP colleagues to identify the most common plants used by the Maasai for medicinal purposes and to document their current conservation status. I planned field visits and scheduled interviews and focus groups, which we conducted inside traditional huts or under trees. As people spoke, I took notes fast and furiously about the plants the villagers spoke about, how they prepared them as medicines, and what maladies they prevented or cured. The information often came so quickly I had to interrupt and ask people to repeat themselves, so that I properly understood what they were sharing.

Back in my office in town, I waded through everything I had collected, working with my British colleague to match up the Maa names with the plant samples that had been identified by a botanical research center and labeled with their Latin names. As I worked to create nicely structured tables to present the information, I noticed something puzzling. Some individual plants were used to treat many different ailments, and some ailments could be treated by an array of different plants.

This confused me enough that I organized another visit to Enguiki village in Maasailand, where I went on a plant walk with an elder Maasai medicine woman. Determined to crack the code, I briefed Sululu on what I was trying to discover so he could translate as precisely as possible for me.

On a hike up Monduli Mountain, in a forest reserve that was abundant with medicinal plants, I followed an elder woman as she moved gracefully and surprisingly quickly through the tall grasses and shrub land. There was no defined trail. Eventually, she stopped and spoke at length about a particular plant, *olamuriaki* (*Carissa edulis*). She explained it could be used for many ailments and that it worked very well. For some, it was especially effective in treating malaria, although others responded better to medicine made from different plants. When I asked if she always collected her own plant medicines when she was working with a patient, she said earlier in her life she had always collected her own plants from the forest, but she confessed that now, since she was getting older, she sometimes sent young warriors to collect the plants she needed.

Her name was Siaety, and she told Sululu she recognized me as a healer as well—which I appreciated. She spoke very openly about how she worked with clients. She always talked at length with them, she said, about their family history, learning about events of the recent past and current issues and complaints. During the long discussion she would tap into sensations in her own body and reflect internally on what she believed was occurring with the patient. Specific plants would then begin to come to her awareness, and she would "talk" to them.

As she walked through the forest in search of the plants her patient needed, she would let the conversation she had had with her patient reverberate in her consciousness. She would feel the patient's symptoms in her own body and silently converse with the plants to get their advice. "I ask the plants I pass which one will help," she said. "They answer me. The plants know you, spiritually, especially the ones you have used before."

I thought to myself, "Wow! *This* is intuition." At the beginning of my time in Maasailand I had been concerned that plant medicine was given willy-nilly to sick children and adults, having been immersed in the scientific method so long and knowing how active ingredients are isolated and tested in a laboratory setting. But I soon discovered that the knowledge of plant medicine in Maasai communities came from intense historical experience. Over centuries, herbalists and healers worked hard to be the bridge between nature's medicine growing on their lands and the patients who could return to health with the plant medicines' help. The Maasai healers' capacity to *listen* to plants and to patients was their laboratory.

SUGGESTED PRACTICE

Knowing that food is medicine, especially fruits and vegetables, take some time to tap into your awareness and listen for a particular fruit or vegetable that may be "talking" to you. Could it contain vitamins and minerals that your body is craving for better health?

SHEEP AND CANCER

From the back of my Suzuki, a sheep let out a loud *"baaa!"* I jumped—I was not accustomed to hearing that sound while driving. Luckily, Sululu was at the wheel and we were making our way down the dry and dusty road from Arusha toward the village of Mkonoo. In the United States, this would be considered a hiking trail at best, but I had become accustomed to traveling on such "roads," although I still didn't enjoy getting tossed around like a rag doll. Poor Tanya, poor sheep. We were on our way to visit Sululu's uncle.

Four years before, Mzee Kipara—his name means "the bald one"—had been diagnosed with prostate cancer, which had metastasized. He had stayed at KCMC hospital in Moshi town for a few months, under the advice of his son, a lab technician there, and was given doses of chemotherapy. Not accustomed to life in the big "city," or modern hospitals, let alone the highly toxic chemicals he was ingesting, the stubborn old man was so distrustful of the treatment he ultimately insisted on leaving the hospital and going home to his Maasai village. No one tried to stop him because the staff at the hospital presumed he didn't have long to live.

When he returned to his home in Mkonoo, he immediately relaxed. He asked his sons and nephews to bring him a sheep periodically—one that was nice and fat—as well as several medicinal plant roots traditionally used by his people. It was Sululu's turn to take his uncle a sheep, and I had patiently waited in the car while he negotiated at the local market.

Now we were only a few kilometers from Kipara's boma, and I

began to consider that we were driving this bleating sheep to its impending slaughter, but perhaps we were also helping save a man's life. Once a fairly strict vegetarian, I learned when you had very little else to eat, and only killed an animal after you had told it how appreciative you were, eating cow, goat, and sheep meat was a blessing. Eating with compassion took on a whole new meaning for me.

When we arrived at the *boma*, we were greeted with a warm welcome. After lengthy greetings, hugs, and singing, we settled onto our tripod wooden stools to speak with the *mzee*. The old man had met me before and remembered my interest in Maasai medicine. He could not wait to tell me how he was outsmarting those doctors in Moshi with the traditional medicine he knew he needed to get better. He described to me the horrible feeling he had had in the hospital room. The place was cold and full of metal and plastic. He missed his mud-and-dung hut with its thatch roof and the warm fire that always kept it warm. He missed his wives and children. And he missed the sounds of nature.

Kipara explained how the sheep we brought would last a while. He would consume every bit of it, except for its eyes—the Maasai don't eat the eyes because they believe they are windows to the animal's soul. He would make a soup from the sheep's fat and mix into it many medicinal plant roots that are soluble in fat. The soup was rebuilding his strength, he said—he could *feel* it, strength that would kill off the cancer cells in his body. He was also very careful to rest, he said, taking it very easy and respecting the illness that was attacking his body was the most important part of his life at this moment. He had to be patient.

Kipara's medicinal soup contained more than twenty species

of plants, including *orkokola, olamuriaki,* and *orkonil.* Some plants were very difficult to obtain because they only grew in specific regions of the country, but extended family members had been dispatched to collect the medicine for their "father." Kipara had discussed his condition with other elder healers who had experience with similar illnesses, and together they had created a customized blend of plant medicines specifically for him. This team effort is always central to Maasai healing. More than simply sending prayers to the patient, family and friends actively participate in the healing process, bringing focused intention and attention to the health of the beloved elder now in his nineties.

Kipara consumed the sheep meat and medicinal soup every day for two months. By then he was able to stand up and walk for the first time in almost a year. "The plant medicines' main purpose was to clear out bad things from Kipara's body," Sululu explained to me, "from the blood and urine. After everything was cleared, Kipara's own strength, his *eishiwo,* took over and brought him back to life."

Mzee Kipara ultimately lived five years following his cancer diagnosis at the town hospital, where doctors had given him just two months to live.

5.

Staying Clean and Clear

WALKING IT OUT

While Freud put people on the couch to sort out pressing issues of the mind, the Maasai take to the earth. Men walk long distances, talking to each other as they go, and traveling to speak with their godfathers, *olage'lie* or *enage'lie*. Women similarly walk and talk to each other, sharing from the heart, typically while collecting firewood or water. A development worker once told me he had just announced to a group of women the establishment of a new well, which would mean they no longer would have to walk a long distance to collect water. The women looked at each other, then asked in dismay, "Why you do this? Now when are we going to have time to talk with each other?" Maasai women discuss a wide array of topics, often about how to deal with men, their husbands, and relatives. These heart-to-heart conversations, in which they speak and listen without judgment, keep both men and women clean and clear of emotional baggage.

When a Maasai has a problem, he or she is taught during initiation to adulthood that you do not blurt out your troubles to just anybody. You have to reach out to the right person and let this person know there is a serious issue you want to discuss. When this person agrees to be your confidant, it's important not to wait long to begin the conversation, because issues that are not discussed can quickly become toxic to the body and the mind. Almost invariably, the person on the receiving end listens compassionately with undivided attention, empathizing without taking on the trauma and drama itself, and playing a vital role in the problem's resolution.

The concept of cleansing is central to Maasai medicine—cleaning the digestive system, the cardiovascular system, and the nervous system, using plant-based medicine to physically clean, and verbal and non-verbal medicine to wash the mind and spirit. Creating and nurturing catharsis can either *become* the cure itself, or the first step that leads the unwell person to further medication. Cleansing the body-mind-spirit is a prerequisite for regaining health in the Maasai world, as it is in most traditional wellness systems.

I have practiced "walking it out" Maasai-style for years. I remember being in Seattle a few years back and meeting an old friend for lunch. Over delicious Caribbean soul food we caught up about jobs, family, mutual friends, and current affairs and told some great stories. When we got to the topic of a personal issue I was grappling with, I suggested we move the venue to the beach, and take a long walk along Puget Sound.

This friend was an *olage'lie* for me, a wise elder, and I truly valued his advice. I could sense that sharing my whole story with him so he could understand my distress was going to be emotionally heavy. It would be much easier to talk outside in nature, with the wind and the waves taking my words away after I had spoken them. I knew from experience that giving voice to thoughts and emotions that were no longer serving me would help send them on their way, and my friend wholeheartedly agreed.

It was a rare, partly sunny June day. The air was still quite cool; the breeze was strong, becoming windy. The view of the sound, as always, was beautiful. It was the perfect location to tell a dark story, and I asked my friend how much time we had, so I could gauge where to begin.

"An hour, more, whatever we need," he said, "I am here for you. Start where you think the story begins."

As we walked along the Puget Sound beach, my friend listened intently. Now and then, he would ask me a question in order to clarify something I said. Or he would ask me to jump ahead. I could tell he *knew* where the story was going, not because he was a mind-reader, but because he recognized some of his own experience, and of others close to him, in the journey I was describing—the human condition being at once so personal and so universal.

When my story reached the present moment, my friend responded by telling me a story from his own life. We had been talking about committed relationships and my disappointment with a romantic partner. My *olage'lie* revealed to me that over forty years before he had expressed to his own father his fear of getting married on the evening before his own wedding. He told me his father spoke very sternly to him and said that while his fear was understandable—given what a treasure his bride was and what strength and courage it would take to keep her—he should never show his fear to her. He encouraged his son to become a man foremost by *enjoying* the journey of marriage with his new wife. If problems arose, he asked his son to bring them to him.

The sun was setting and I felt relieved, affirmed, happy. Some of the residual doubts I had been harboring about my decision to end a distressing relationship literally disappeared into the wind and the sea—and I felt free.

SUGGESTED PRACTICE

When a particular incident in your life hits you hard and you can't seem to shake it off, consider reaching out to a friend, family member, or trusted advisor and suggest taking a walk.

Plan enough time. Choose a location in nature.

Tell your story fully. Get it all out.

Storytelling as therapy is an art form. Let's imagine that you tell a trusted friend or therapist your problem is something that happened to you that morning—perhaps you had a fight with your son. But that day's conflict is only the most up-to-the-minute scene in a performance that lasts a lifetime. In order to understand both the argument and the way forward, you have to begin in a previous scene. Choose one that feels relevant. As you tell your story you can feel internally whether the story is making sense. Pay attention to the reaction of your listener.

Celebrate the clearing when it is complete, the visceral release of baggage. Depending on the issue, of course, it may take more than one pass through—more than a single deep sharing with a trusted friend—to get completely clear.

FASTING FOR A BLACK HEART

I asked Sululu whether the Maasai ever fast like people in other cultures do, but I felt silly even before my words were out. I knew how difficult it was for Maasai to have enough food simply to survive; why in the world would they consciously refrain from eating? Yet Sululu's answer truly surprised me.

"We do fast. When a person feels *erok olndau*, which means 'having a black heart,' the body becomes too full-up with everything, from food to thoughts to other toxins built up from relationship problems and other stressful events. The digestion starts to shut down. Nothing gets processed properly and there is no room to consume anything else. There is no choice but to fast.

"We don't eat anything for twenty-four hours or more. We leave the body to work on itself. We let it decide what it wants to do without forcing anything else into it. We just relax and let the natural processing and digestion take over. Your body tells you what to do. Sometimes we drink some medicinal tea to move the digestion along. If there is a lot to clean out, we will vomit or have diarrhea. It is often after all has been cleaned out that we then know what is going on. Either we ate some bad food, someone has died, or we haven't made peace with somebody."

ORLPUL, STRENGTHENING BODY MIND SPIRIT

Going on *orlpul* in Maasai culture is the ultimate experience of renewal and rejuvenation. It is akin to a spa retreat in that participants go to a sacred place and cut themselves off from news from the outside world, cleansing their bodies and going into the forest to concentrate on getting strength deep in the womb of Mother Nature.

Men, women, children, and warriors all take part in *orlpul*, the name referring both to forest or bushland and to the ritual itself. During an *orlpul*, a group of Maasai people come together to experience the cleansing effects of living off the environment, living in the wild and eating a healing soup containing meat, fat, blood, and herbal medicines. For warriors, called *ilmurran*, *orlpul* is a ritual that allows them the ability to reap the benefits of the forest—spiritual power, fierceness, and physical strength that makes them ready for battle, whether literally or figuratively. Children, women, and older men attend *orlpul* with the intention of re-building their bodies before and after major crises in their lives or for the general maintenance of physical health and well-being.

My friend Leboy Ololtimbau, a Maasai man from Monduli who is about thirty, first went on *orlpul* when he was five. "I am the first born son of my father," he told me. "My dad would like to take me on *orlpul* because he really loved me and wanted to teach me things. Of course I don't really remember everything he was trying to teach me when I was so young. It was a hard time because I didn't really want the medicinal soup, I wanted to drink milk! We are supposed to go to *orlpul* before circumcision because you know you are going to lose a lot of blood. I did this when I was twenty-one. We took four cows and went for three months."

I asked Leboy if there were other reasons to go on *orlpul*. "Yes, to treat sickness and to get strong, and also to relax after working hard all year. The purpose is to strengthen yourself and treat yourself so you can protect your family and community. We have different kinds of *orlpul*, a treatment *orlpul*, and a warrior *orlpul* and an elder *orlpul*, *larpayani*. On elder *orlpul*, we as young people are asked to go along to help prepare the meat, do the work. The elders teach us during those times.

"*Eramatata*, treatment *orlpul*, happens when someone is sick. Usually, one person who is sick goes with five to seven healthy people. I remember when I had a broken foot, my father helped heal me. He took me to *orlpul*, he tied sheep skin to hold my leg in place. He gave me medicine and made me rest."

I asked Leboy how a site is chosen for *orlpul*. "Some people use dreams. Especially the elders, they see sacred places in their dreams. The place should feel peaceful, with trees nearby to protect you."

Every *orlpul* site must be near water, which is important for preparing medicinal soups; medicinal trees must also be close at hand, and plenty of shade is vital to prevent the meat from spoiling too quickly. "Sometimes we don't go back to the same place for up to three years," he said. We say that people have been there and we don't know what they have done there, what needed to be cleaned, so it is better to leave it."

An *orlpul* site is always constructed within natural clearings in the forest or bush. Each *orlpul* has a day area, *oleng'oti*, which is also used for cooking, and a sleeping area, *enkirragata*, which is protected by a circular fence composed of acacia thorn branches to protect those sleeping inside from animals outside. Within *enkirragata*, the bedding is made from camphor leaves, *oleleshua* and *osendu*, that repel insects and retain heat. In both the day and sleeping area sites, fires are tended continually.

Once a site has been prepared and the participants have gathered, no one is allowed to enter or leave. The enclosure becomes a haven for those taking part in *orlpul*, keeping them safe from animals on the outside and creating a sacred space on the inside.

"Sometimes we go on *orlpul* without telling people. It is a secret among a group of us. Especially if we have to steal the cows for it." I understood that part of the healing that happens on *orlpul* is the result of sacrifices of both time and resources that people make in order to participate.

"We have places we choose that are cooler during the hot months, and warmer areas we go to during the cold months. Sometimes you just walk along and feel this is the right place for *orlpul*. The temperature is middle, just right. Not too hot, not too cold. During the rainy season, we don't often go, because the meat will get rotten too quickly. However, if someone is very sick, they can't wait, and have to go during the rains. Near my house is a big cave; that is a good place to go if there is rain. It provides shelter. You can sleep in there, and even stand up. There are some people who can feel some places are really good for healing, in the same way as there are some people who can feel where a lion has passed.

"Parents will give cows and goats for the *orlpul*. We all stay together the night before and leave in the middle of the night. We don't want the women to see where we are going. It is a secret for men, for warriors. It can be a three, or five hour walk, sometimes a whole day of walking. Together with the livestock, we travel with a pot, cups, a bucket for water and knives.

"The first days we prepare the site. We make a circle of

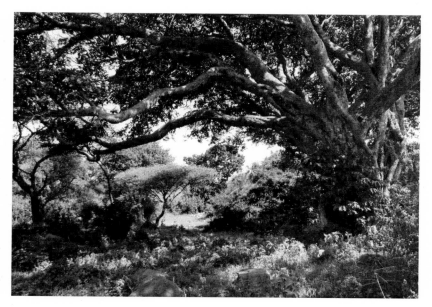

An ideal site for an orlpul

branches and then we prepare the places to sleep. We make the
fire, collect the medicinal plants. It is a lot of work to collect all the
medicine. We divide the jobs; say, two people collect the medicine,
two people cook the meat, two people make the soup.

"You can drink the soup up to three times a day. The soup is
made of water, medicinal plants, and the bones, tongue, and hooves
of the animal. We put the blood somewhere, sometimes in the
soup. We put the fat of the animal in the soup because we want the
soup to be fatty, it makes the plants less bitter. Also, if you feel dry,
the fatty soup makes you feel less dry. I drink fat often, if I eat in
town something that makes me feel dry or if the food inside gets

stuck and won't go down. You can diarrhea from eating or drinking the fat. It helps move the stuff through the body.

"At *orlpul* you can poo a lot. There are plants that are given to people to help them poo. To stop it if it is too much you give sour milk, or yogurt. It stops the diarrhea. It is very nice; you become, how do I say, not heavy. You feel light."

The fusion of water, fat, meat, bones, medicines, and blood in the medicinal soup, *emotorik*, cleans the body completely. As uninviting as vomiting or diarrhea sound, they hold the key to emptying, cleansing, and reinvigorating the body. A woman who has attended several *orlpuls* told me, "I felt strong and energized. Before, I had a hard time climbing up the mountain, but I ran up the hill easily! These medicines last a few days, after which time you actually feel better."

Songs, prayer, and meditation are important during *orlpul*. "We have one person appointed to open the day and close the day," Leboy said. "He has high-capacity thinking and knows how to bless. He opens and closes the door of the circle. We have special songs we sing for *orlpul*; we sing whenever we feel the need to sing. I have never been on *orlpul* when someone gets sick, never. Everyone gets strong and light. We have a competition sometimes who can eat the most meat. We have very bitter plants that help us digest; the digestion really runs fast. You don't drink water, only water with medicine. If you drink the water you make people lazy and tired. The water needs to be mixed with something that helps you digest.

"The meat can be stored in a little house made of branches for a couple of days. These branches have anti-bacterial power and help keep away the flies. We have some medicine that makes people cry, until all the tears are out. *Esenyi* does this. It washes their spirit.

"Traditionally, women went on *orlpul* to get their strength after they had a baby. They prefer to go with elders, and a husband can take his wife and his son. The women always stay separately from men; they don't eat together.

"Something very special I like about *orlpul* is the *eilata nan-yokie*, the red fat. You take five kilos of fat from an old bull and mix with nine different plants, and water. The fat is cooked early in the morning, for an hour. Then *olorien* is put on the fire and heated and then goes in the fat mixture—it smells so nice! It is making my mind go back there. I love it. The nine plants are *orltima, achani onyokie, oremiti, orkokola, asanagururii, orkiloriti, ormukutan, olorien, olesupeni*. Some, you use the leaves, others the roots, or bark. It has to be a big pot, because everybody likes it! You make it in the middle of *orlpul*. It is red in color. I really like this *eilata nanyokie*; the taste is very nice."

The Maasai believe that the medicines consumed in *orlpul* facilitate the cleansing of the body and that the large quantities of meat and fat consumed rebuild bodily strength by promoting the production of blood. The quantity and quality of one's blood, they believe, is the chief determinant of overall health.

Scientific research demonstrates that the plants consumed in *orlpul* help improve digestion and aid in eliminating accumulated toxins. As an oil, the herbalized fat works as a laxative, moving gastrointestinal contents out through the colon. The procedure is similar to *virechana*, purgation, in the Ayurvedic medicine system.

"Also, we leave some meat for our animal friends," Leboy added, "for the lions and hyena—like the cow's large stomach. We also carry roasted meat for the young boys herding cows, and for the ladies. When you get back home from *orlpul*, all the bomas collect milk for you. We mix sour milk with blood to open the stomach to agree with other food. After that you brush your teeth, wash your body. We walk around the bomas, singing, celebrating. It is a nice ceremony."

During a traditional *orlpul*, the Maasai stay in the sacred forest retreat for days, even up to a month or more. People sleep when they need to sleep, eat when they are hungry, and sing and dance together often. Sharing and storytelling help heal psychological wounds and disconnections and facilitate general bonding that restores the soul. When Maasai people come off an *orlpul*, they are strong, healthy, and ready to re-enter the world.

"When there is one cow left, and the *orlpul* feels it is coming to an end, we report back to the *bomas* that we are finishing. The mamas at home prepare the milk, the yogurt, the *olkaria*—red clay—and necklaces with good smelling plants. As warriors, we have a special song we sing twice a day for four days before we come out."

> *Papa lai otoishe mekintoki ajo lanyorro tejoki engukuu.*
> My lovely Daddy, don't call me beloved son, call me Imaginary.
> *Najulukunya "Oletupe" naning'o ake toonyorin ejoke.*
> Who usually keep a long hair like imaginary, or like savages. Who you may know from war-like breathing.

Yenyeyenye nejo Olang'oni osira ekume akeyeu.

Trotting, ha! ha! And I said I need a colored bull with a brand on its mouth.

Oingwa lidosero odung'o ekume lorkumbene lesuya.

From the woodland, like a corridor to paradise, of a man known as Olesuya.

Yeyo!

Yayo lai natoishe. Mekitoki ajo lang'ututu tejoki.

My lovely Mum, don't call me beloved son, call me Imaginary.

Eng'ukuu najulukunya "Oletupe" naning'o ake toonyorin.

Who usually keep a long hair like imaginary, or like savages. Who you may know from war-like breathing.

Ejake yenyeyenye nejo alang'oni osira ekume akewu.

Trotting, ha! ha! And I said I need a colored bull with a brand on its mouth.

Oingwa lidosero odung'o ekume lorkumbene lesuya.

From the woodland, like a corridor to paradise, of a man known as Olesuya.

Red clay, called *olkaria,* has been used by the Maasai for centuries to remove impurities and dead skin cells. After a strong cleansing, toxins move to the surface of the skin and the *olkaria* scrubs them off completely. It is considered a beautiful adornment for the body, and it softens and smooths the texture of the skin.

I asked Leboy if he still goes on *orlpul.* "Yes. But because I am really busy, I can't go very often. During the times between *orlpul,*

I miss it. But I drink a lot of prevention medicine in between."

A comprehensive study by McGill University in Toronto examined nineteen plant food additives used by the Maasai of Kenya and Tanzania in relation to their possible role in lowering cholesterol. The findings were startling. Eighty-two percent of the food additives screened contained chemicals that definitively lower cholesterol, including polyphenols, phytosteroids, water soluble dietary fibers, antioxidants, flavonoids, and saponins. It is very possible they play a major role in lowering the rates of coronary heart diseases among indigenous Maasai, who continue to live in rural areas, eat heavy red-meat diets, and practice their traditional systems of health care.

Sululu, of course, was not surprised by the findings. "The plant medicine works partly because of the active ingredients and partly because of trust. The medicine works best when it is part of a process—your interaction with your people, in nature with *Engai*, when you build up to a point in your story where it makes sense to take the medicine and how to take the medicine in the right way. You heal."

SUGGESTED PRACTICE

You don't have to live in a Maasai village to experience
the benefits of this approach to health and wellbeing.
An *orlpul* experience can be created anywhere that has
a pristine and sacred natural environment, nourishing and strength-giving food, and a group of people to
share the experience.

Next time you feel particularly weak, create your own
orlpul.

Take time to prepare. Who would you invite to join
you? What food would you prepare? Plan for others
to take over your responsibilities during your time in
orlpul.

Consider using a gentle cleansing program made
of herbal preparations that have been scientifically
formulated.

During your *orlpul,* sing meaningful songs together
and tell stories that help you focus on re-connecting
with your deepest collectively held values, beliefs,
intentions, and desires. Take the time for heartfelt
discussion.

Let others know when you are coming back so they
can welcome you and prepare a celebration ceremony.

SPIRITUAL HEALERS, *LAIBONIS*

Ikweti kake miilanyi esipata.
You can keep running a lot but you can't hide
from the truth.

Un-wellness and disease in traditional Maasai culture is addressed
first at home, with self-care and assistance from those closest to
you. If, after taking plant medicine, or walking it out, or going on
orlpul, someone still is not feeling well, it may be time to bring
in the services of a *laiboni,* a spiritual healer. A true, experienced
laiboni uses ritual divination to identify the root cause of illness.
During a session, the spiritual healer creates a field of attention,
intention, and coherence between himself, the patient, and the
patient's ancestors that allows the healer to see unhealthy patterns
that can be transformed. He then prescribes specific plant medicines, either to consume internally or to use externally to cleanse
or protect the patient's spirit, or aura, as well as suggesting affir-
mations and prayers for the patient to repeat.

In the same way that some Maasai are called to the profession
of herbalist, others' purpose in life is to become spiritual leaders,
laibonis. In traditional Maasai culture, it is most often men who
receive the special gifts, or spiritual talents, from *Engai,* which
are passed on from father to son. These gifts enable *laibonis* to
serve their tribe by foretelling future events, helping their communities to make the best collective decisions, and helping people
work through spiritual crises. Being a *laiboni* is a deeply respected
position, and because of their prophetic abilities and knowledge

of medicinal healing, people often depend on *laibonis* for advice regarding major events, spiritual ceremonies, and preparation of medicines for treating various types of ailments. Because it is a profession requiring great experience and knowledge, a son becomes his father's apprentice while he is still young.

Laibonis use two main tools to do their work: they interpret their patients' dreams and they read the energetic arrangement of pebbles, bones, and stones that they throw from a buffalo horn or gourd. The throwing of bones and stones activates the connection between the healer and his patient, and the work of a good *laiboni* in Maasai culture parallels that of good spiritual healers around the world.

The journey to get to a *laiboni*'s place of work can take days because many live in remote areas in the bush. With Sululu, I have visited many *laibonis* throughout Maasailand and have been treated by them. The first time I sat in front of a *laiboni*, I tested him. I did not say anything about who I was or what I wanted. I was curious to see just how good he was at reading me. He asked me to spit into his calabash full of stones and then threw them onto a sweater I had handed to him. I watched as he studied, then began to move some of the stones into groupings. Finally, he began to ask me questions. "Is it true that you have a new job with a chance to influence a lot of people?" It was true. I was amazed.

When he continued to astonish me with his insights into my life, I eventually thought I understood how he did so. It was as if he were holding a mirror in front of me. My story was emerging through the interaction between me and the healer. With every insight he offered, he asked very humbly if I agreed or disagreed, then used my response to move the totality of my life-story that was emerging in the proper direction. Very quickly, he uncovered surprising details of my personal history, including those that most significantly contributed to my current state of affairs.

With every patient, Sululu explained, the *laiboni* helps locate the crux of a particular problem, targets it, then prescribes a way to move ahead, through elimination techniques and neutralization. The special gift of a *laiboni* is *eyelounoto*, the ability to be conscious of a patient's past, present, and future all in one moment.

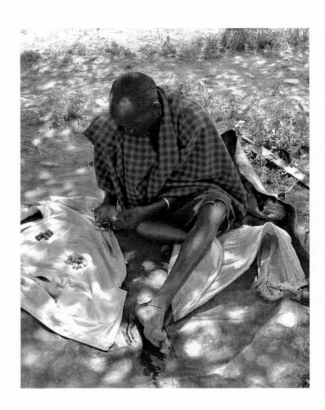

A laiboni at work

A great deal of healing works on the energetic level. Elimination involves some type of sacrifice—the decision to surrender something in your life you thought you could not live without. By giving it up, you can move forward. In Maasai culture, the most common sacrifice is the surrender of a cow, goat, or sheep—the culture's most valuable possessions. Neutralization involves the use of protective plants that are ground into a powder, then added to a warm-water bath. The patient bathes with single-minded awareness that she is literally "washing her spirit." Wearing protective plants as necklaces is also common during the time one works with a *laiboni*.

Neither expert practitioners of plant medicine or spirit healers charge for their services, but it is universally understood that a patient will give the healer a gift as soon as she is well. In traditional Maasailand, this is almost invariably livestock; in urban areas, money is given to the healer as a thanksgiving. Everyone understands that in order for healers to continue their work, these gifts are essential.

The Maasai do not believe in witchcraft, sorcery, or devil worship. I quickly learned while living and working in Maasailand that because the environment is so harsh, it is vital for people to have a close connection with *Engai*, Mother Nature, and with each other. The Maasai believe that your current state of wellness depends on your history and the health of your relationships. The only way to move forward on a pathway is to not repeat mistakes, but to learn from them.

"A mistake is only a mistake if it is repeated," Sululu assured me, explaining that a *laiboni* asks you to give details about your family history and personal patterns of behavior in order to understand the causes of your *dis*-ease. Only then can he prescribe medicine to neutralize the flow of negativity that is keeping you from moving forward on a new healthy path. When everyone in a community is ready to cut the cord of unhealthy patterns, a ritual is organized to mark the turning point. Traditionally, livestock were sacrificed—the killing of a cow was the ultimate sacrifice. That kind of loss is not easy to forget, and it works in profound ways to push you in a new direction.

Sometimes, sacrifices take the form of burning material possessions, or throwing important items into rivers or oceans, letting the water take them away. Once a ritual is complete, the problem or issue no longer exists. "That file has been deleted," Sululu explained, enjoying his very modern metaphor.

SUGGESTED PRACTICE

If you are suffering from chronic stress and stress-related illnesses that have not responded well to other medicine, consider finding a healer skilled at mind-body-spirit work.

Find a skilled healer who you trust and feel comfortable with.

Work with your healer to understand patterns in your life that are no longer serving you.

Identify together a meaningful sacrifice you can make to push you forward. Give away an important possession, donating money or time to a cause larger than yourself, cut or shave your hair.

Create a ritual around the sacrifice and the death of the "old you." Bring in others who will support the "new you."

Celebrate your progress.

MOVING FROM HEAD TO HEART

I had been practicing yoga for two years before I moved to Tanzania, and in 1998 in Seattle, I was a regular student at a lovely yoga studio near my home in the Greenlake area of the city. My body-mind seemed to move into a wonderful state of bliss after each class that was led by a wonderful instructor named Mary. In those days, my regular yoga practice was of vital help to me as I navigated the stormy waters of writing, then defending my Ph.D. dissertation. At each yoga class, I was able to move out of my head, giving my overtaxed mind a brief respite from philosophical debates, and instead focus on keeping my body in line and in balance. Spending most of each day either in front of students or at my computer made me feel like I was a walking and talking head—but yoga helped me reconnect to the rest of me.

When I told Mary that I was planning to head to East Africa to live and work, she said, "I will join you there one day. But I am not ready yet." Mary is African-American and explained that she was mustering the courage to explore the faraway home of her ancestors. She knew going to Africa would be an emotional journey and she needed to be prepared. But she was excited for me.

I asked if she could design a yoga sequence that I could practice privately in Tanzania because I knew I wouldn't be encountering yoga studios there. While I felt comfortable practicing yoga in a class setting, I had not yet moved from being a student, guided by a teacher, to practicing on my own.

Mary wanted to know my birthday, because she combines astrological information with her practice of yoga and massage. Knowing the tendencies within a personality type based on birth date helps her to understand how a client moves and uses her body.

When the day of my departure was fast approaching and I still hadn't heard from Mary, I called her. "Oh, Tanya!" she exclaimed. "I had your whole program made up and then it dawned on me. You will no longer be swimming in the mind-world of academia and American life in the Pacific Northwest. You are going to Africa! The home of the heart. I need to quickly re-work your program so that you will remember you have a head as you move around in the heart world."

I was not entirely sure what she meant by this, but I trusted Mary, so I waited another day to meet with her and learn my yoga sequence for Africa—the home of the heart.

After just a few months in Arusha, I discovered exactly what Mary was talking about. I could literally feel the energy dropping down from my head to my chest, where my heart sits. To this day, I still cannot explain what was physically responsible for this shift—some kind of gravitational pull, or something about the pervasive African culture that encourages your words and actions to come from your heart center, rather than initiating in your mind. Whatever it is, it feels good to me—and I'm a Gemini with an overactive mind.

Many people have spoken to me over the years about this phenomenon, including students and tourists from the west who explain that they feel like they "lose their heads" when they journey to the African continent. Many of them note how emotional the locals are, how passionate they can be—both men and women—and it is refreshing to witness such honest and expressive humanity.

When I began teaching yoga myself in Arusha, then later in Dar es Salaam and Zanzibar, I remembered Mary's words. My students, most of them European immigrants and local Tanzanians working for American and European businesses, universally complained of stress. As I heard their stories, I immediately understood the disconnect they experienced between being based in Tanzania and communicating with business partners overseas. Heads and hearts were not interacting with ease, with productivity, or with peace.

So, I created a yoga sequence as part of my Maasai yoga program specifically for re-connecting head and heart. It has kept me and many of my students in one piece over the years. And it has helped nurture the tremendous combined power of a strong head and a strong heart, working in unison.

Maasai Yoga Asana Series

6.

Maasai Yoga
Asana Series

This sequence includes many poses representing the animals that live together with the Maasai. It is a sequence that helps connect your head to your heart and promotes strength, balance and flexibility. Move into the poses that feel good to you, paying close attention to your mind-body. Remember to breathe naturally and move through the practice as effortlessly as possible.

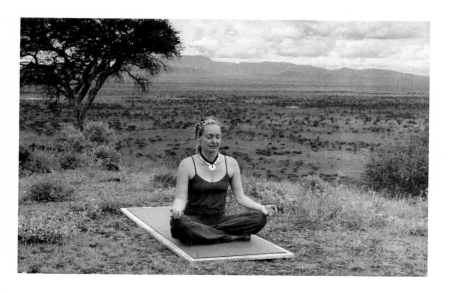

Begin in a cross-legged pose.

Sit comfortably in a cross-legged position. Close your eyes and relax your face, your jaw, your neck and shoulders. Breathe deeply into your belly.

Cow-cat poses.

Slowly open your eyes and come onto your hands and knees. Your hands are below your shoulders, your knees are below your hips. On the inhale, bring your head and tailbone in opposite directions into cow pose. On the exhale, tuck your tailbone and drop your head to come into the cat pose. Repeat this several times then push back into child's pose.

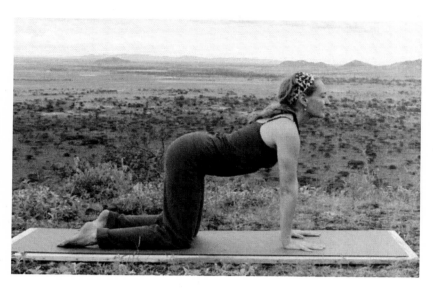

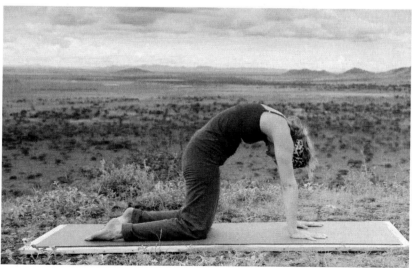

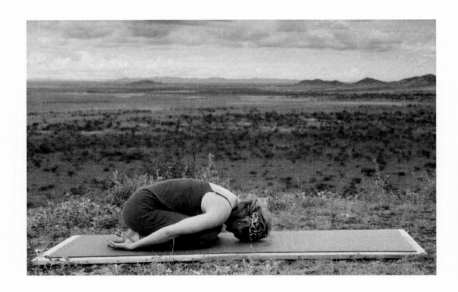

Child's Pose

From your hands and knees, push back to sit on your heels. Rest your forehead on the mat and either keep your arms extended out in front of you or bring your arms along your sides and place your hands outside your ankles with your palms facing up.

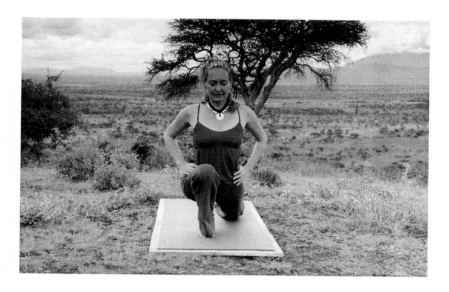

Parrot pose.

Step your right foot forward between your hands, making sure your right knee is in front of the ankle. Keeping your back knee on the mat, place your hands on your hips and breathe, stretching out your thigh. Change legs, placing the left foot forward.

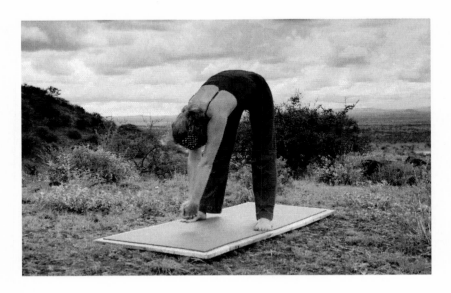

Elephant pose.

Step both feet wide in the center of your mat and bend forward to-wards the earth. Clasp your hands together making an elephant's trunk with your arms. Slowly move you arms, swaying your trunk from side to side. Initiate the movement from your lower back, lubricating your spine. Let your head hang as you move, and keep breathing.

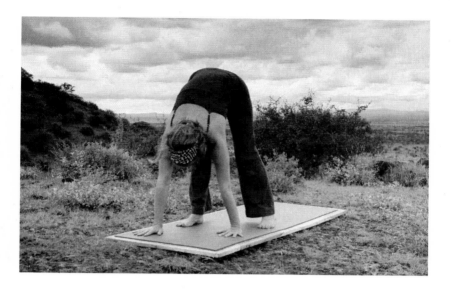

Giraffe pose.

Place your hands on the mat so you are now on four 'legs'. Giraffes walk with their back leg and front leg moving together. So step forward and backwards along your mat, first moving your right side, then left side. Distribute your weight equally and move gracefully, like a giraffe in the bush.

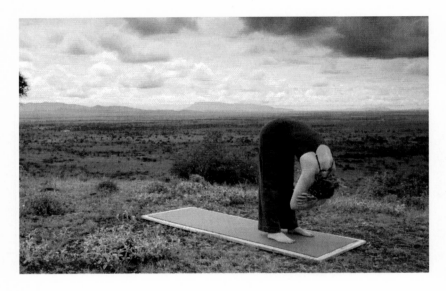

Standing forward bend pose.

Staying in a forward bend with your head relaxed and reaching towards the earth, grab a hold of your opposite elbows with your hands. Breathe and feel your spine lengthen. To come up, bend your knees slightly and slowly roll all the way to stand tall.

Sun Salutations.

Sun salutations honor the sun that shines on us on this earth, giving us energy and light. Each salutation includes 12 poses that link together to form a flowing dance.

Begin standing at the top of your mat, feet hip-width apart. Reach your hands towards the sky then bend over, hands towards your mat. Extend your left leg back bending your right knee into a lunge. Then, step your right foot back to meet the left foot and breathe into your downward dog pose. Move forward into a plank pose, then come all the way down to the mat. Push up into cobra pose. Tuck your toes, lifting your tailbone, push back into downward dog. Keep breathing. Step the left foot forward, keeping the back knee down. Step both feet together into the forward bend. Finish by reaching toward the sky, then bring your palms together in front of your heart. Feel your heart beating. You can repeat this full sun salutation series several times, making it a dance.

(Photographs on the following pages)

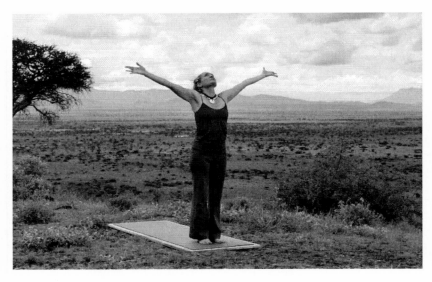

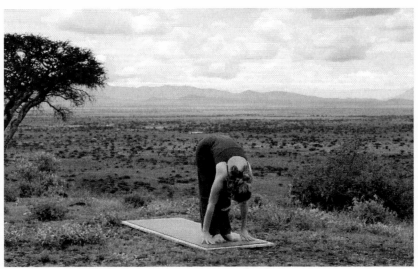

Sun Salutations, 1 – 4

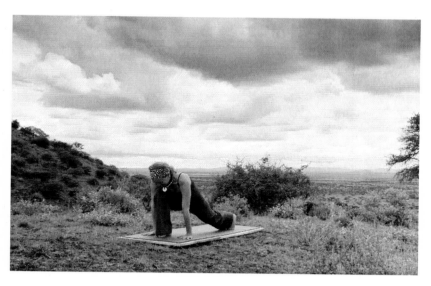

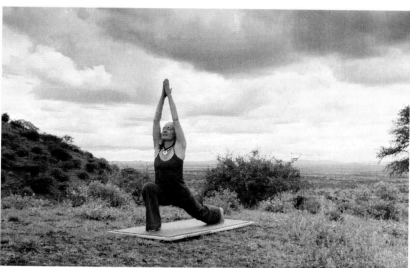

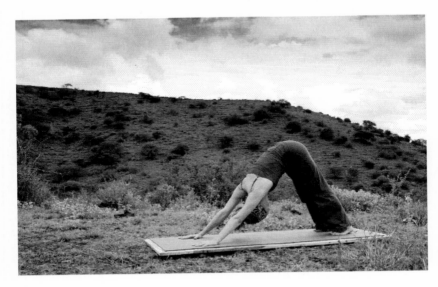

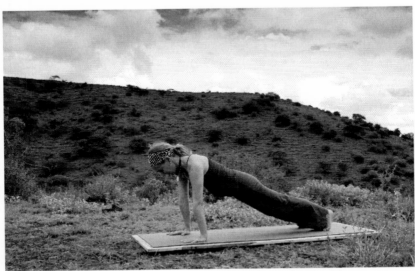

Sun Salutations, 5 – 8

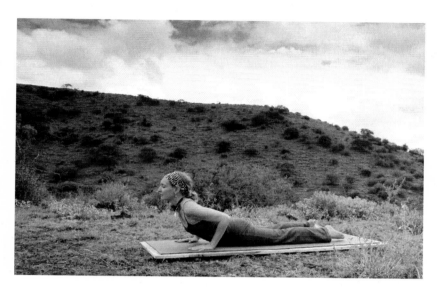

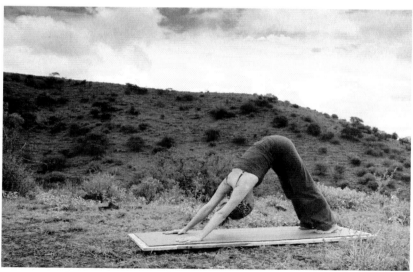

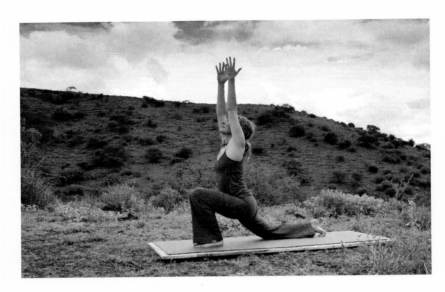

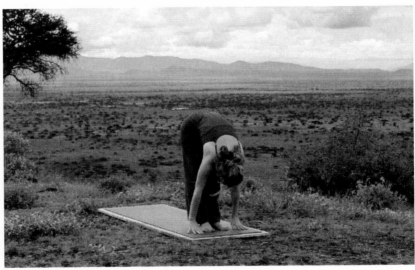

Sun Salutations, 9 – 12

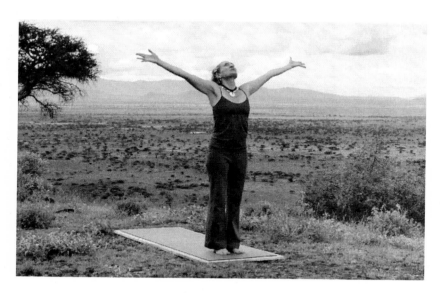

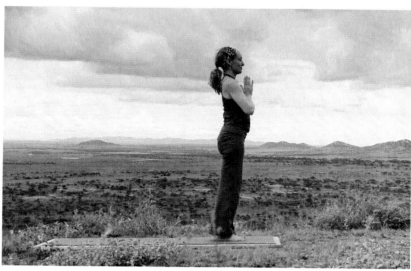

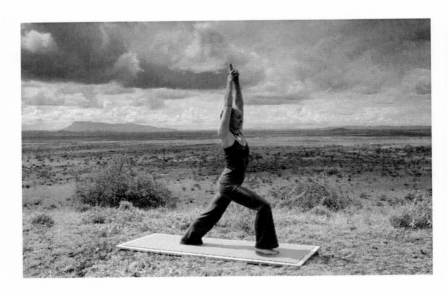

Peaceful Maasai Warrior poses – I, II, III

Begin warrior I pose from standing. Take a big step back with your left leg, placing your left foot down at an angle so that your back heel lines up with your front heel. Reach your arms up, pointing towards the sky. Lunge into your right leg, with your right knee in line with your right ankle. From here, open up into the warrior II pose. Reach your arms in opposite directions, gazing fiercely over the third finger of your right hand. Relax your shoulders, open your chest, and breathe. Come back to warrior I pose, stepping the left foot in slightly, hips straight ahead. Find your balance and slowly come into warrior III pose by shifting your weight forward into your front leg as you lift your back leg so that your arms, torso and back leg are parallel to the earth. Breathe and feel the courage and balance of this pose. Bring your foot down and repeat this peaceful Maasai warrior series on the other side.

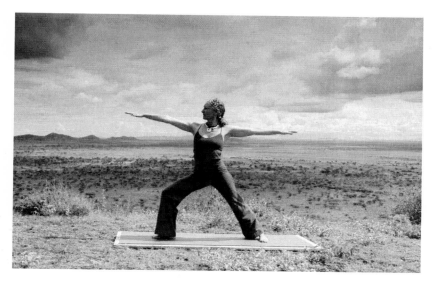

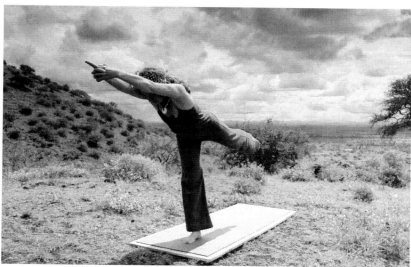

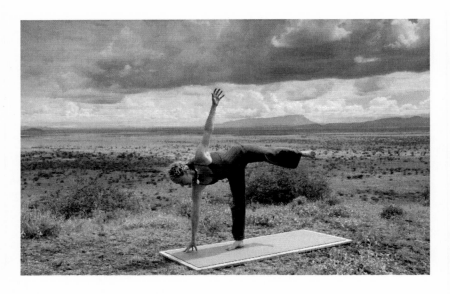

Warrior II into Half Moon pose.

First find your solid warrior II pose. Then place your right hand down on the mat as if you were cupping a tennis ball. Find your balance and then lift your left leg up so it is parallel to the earth. Either stay here, with your left hand on your hip, or you can reach the left hand towards the sky for the full expression of a half moon over the African savannah. Keep breathing. Slowly come up, stepping back to warrior II pose. Repeat on the other side.

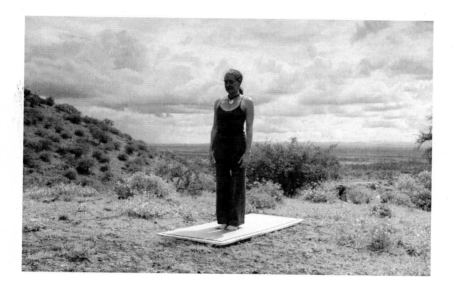

Stand in Mountain Pose and breathe deeply.

Stand with your feet hip-width apart, toes pointing straight ahead, arms by your sides with your fingertips reaching down toward the earth. Close your eyes and feel your balance and your strength.

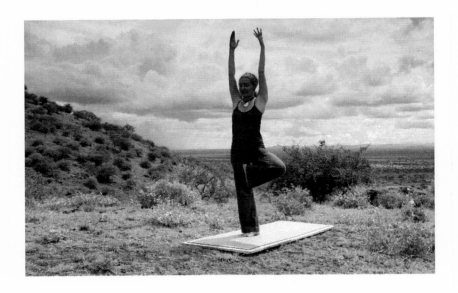

Tree pose.

Rooting your right foot into the earth, bring the left foot up and place it either on your inner thigh, or on your shin. Bring your palms together in front of your chest. You can stay here or you can grow the branches of your tree towards the sun. Maasai boys stand in tree pose when they are herding their cattle, they say it is a balancing pose and very relaxing. Repeat on the other side, rooting your left foot into the earth. Always keep breathing.

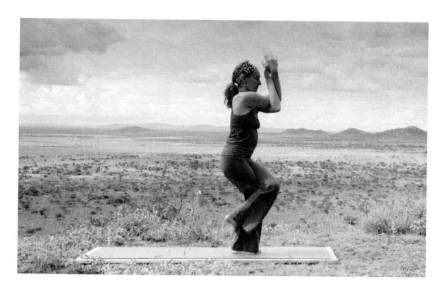

Eagle pose.

From standing, root your right foot into the earth and bring your left leg around the right leg, bending both knees, as if sitting in a chair. Wrap your left arm underneath the right arm and bring your palms to meet each other. Lift your elbows to shoulder height while keeping your shoulders back and down. Breathe deeply. Repeat on the other side. When finished, root both feet into the ground, coming to land back on the earth.

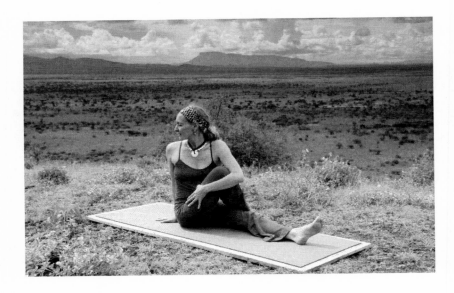

Seated Twist pose.

Gracefully, come back down to sit on your mat, with your legs out straight in front of you. Your spine is straight. Bring your right foot over the left leg and place the foot flat on your mat. Place your right hand a short distance from your right buttock and with your left arm, grab a hold of your right leg. Slowly spiral around your tailbone, visualize making a corkscrew with your spine. Gaze out over your right shoulder. Keep breathing. Slowly unwind and repeat on the other side.

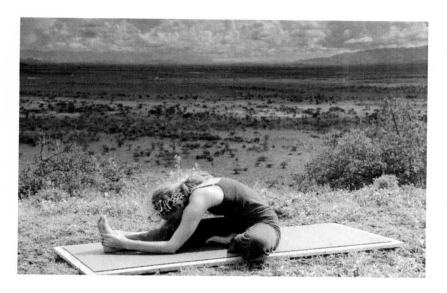

Sitting Tree pose.

Starting from a seated position with both legs straight ahead, bend your left leg and bring your left foot to your thigh. Reach past your right foot to come down over your right leg, as far as you can. With each breath, try and go a little deeper into the pose. Change sides.

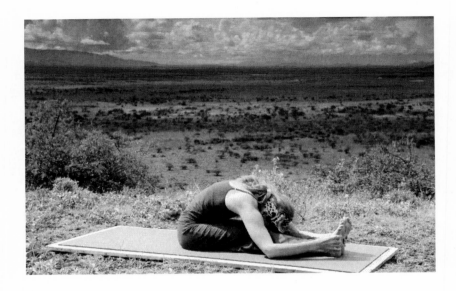

Seated Forward Bend pose.

From a seated position with both legs straight ahead and your spine straight, slowly come down as far as you can, reaching past your toes. Close your eyes and surrender to the breath. Enjoy the stretch as you go deeper with each breath.

Butterfly pose.

From a seated position, bend both knees and bring the soles of your feet together, letting your knees relax to the sides. Slowly bring your head toward your feet while you breathe deeply, lengthening the muscles around your hips and spine. Then, reach your right arm up towards the sky, lubricating your shoulder joints. Change arms, reach the left arm up, making space for your heart and lungs.

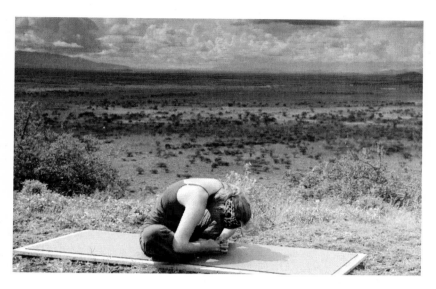

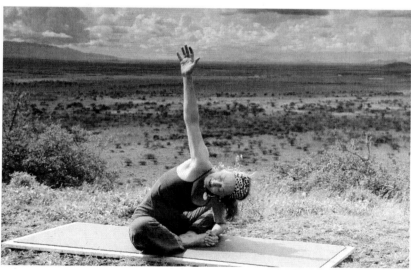

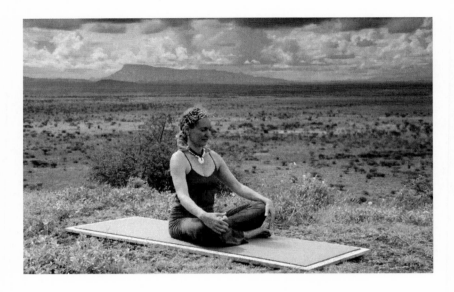

Fire log pose.
Place a bent right leg over bent left leg, as you place logs on
the fire, giving space for air to move through. Keep your spine
straight and breathe into your hips. Relax. Change legs, placing
the left leg over the right.

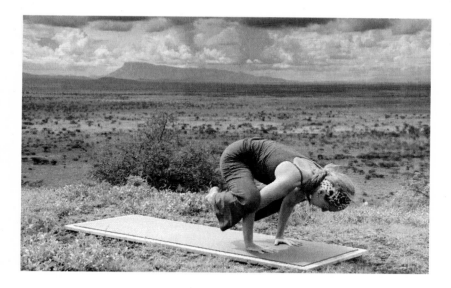

Crane pose.

Start in a squat position. Bring your palms flat onto the mat in front of you, and slowly position your knees on your upper arms, placing weight into your upper body. Either keep your toes on the ground, or move into the full expression of crane pose by finding your balance point and gently lifting your feet off the ground. Bring your toes to touch behind you and keep breathing.

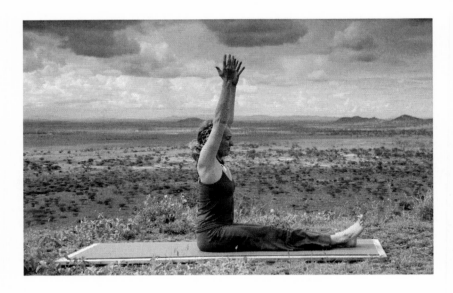

Core strengthening flow.

Start by bringing your legs out in front of you in a seated position on your mat, spine straight. Reach your hands to the sky, and initiating from your belly button, slowly roll to a flat back, arms to your sides. Bring your knees in towards your chest, then reach the feet up towards the sky, and then slowly drop your legs towards the earth. Keep your awareness at initiating your movements from your belly. Bring your knees back into your chest, and then lengthen your whole body along your mat. Keep moving by using your abdominal muscles to bring yourself up, reaching your arms past your feet and coming into a forward bend. Breathe. Flowing back up, gently come roll back to lie flat on your mat. You can repeat this flow several times.

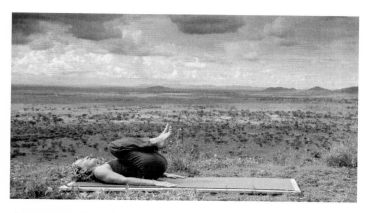

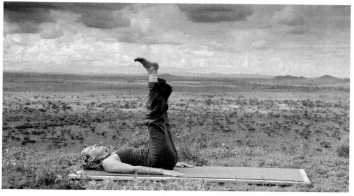

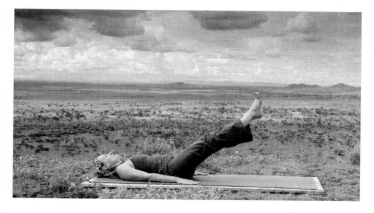

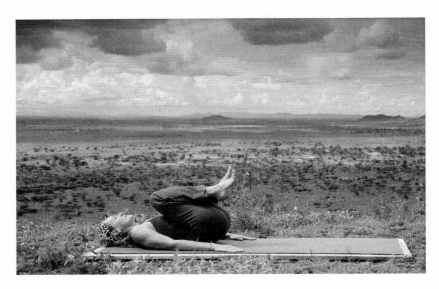

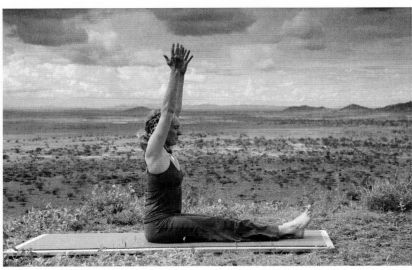

Core strenthening flow continued

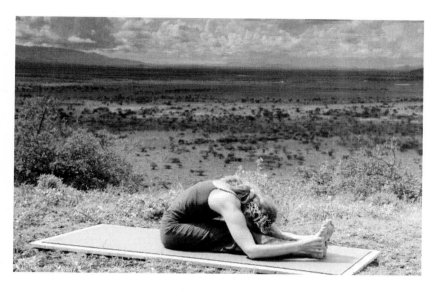

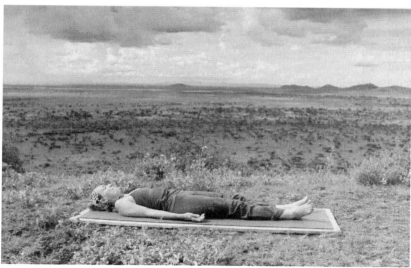

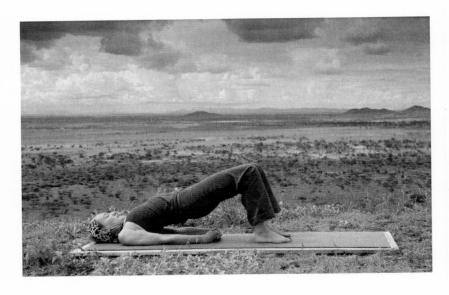

Bridge pose.

Making a bridge from your head to your feet, begin on your back with your legs bent and feet flat on the mat, about hip-distance apart. Pushing into the soles of your feet, knees and toes straight ahead, gently begin lifting your hips towards the sky. You can keep your arms and hands facing down or you can clasp your hands together underneath your body, bringing your shoulders toward one another and your chin gently toward your chest. Breath easily, keeping your jaw nice and relaxed. Come out of this pose slowly, bringing your hips gently back to the earth.

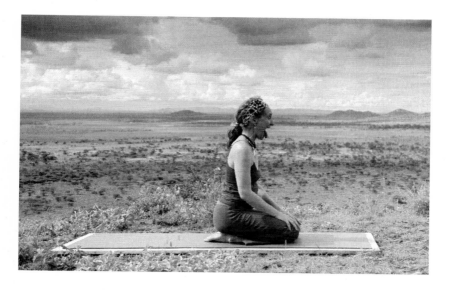

Lion pose.

Now for the king of the jungle, the lion. Sit on your heels and place your hands on your knees, keeping your spine straight. Inhale deeply and close your eyes. On the exhale, stick your tongue out and roar as a lion opening your eyes wide and looking towards the sky. Repeat three times, or more.

Camel pose.

Kneel on your mat with your knees hip-width apart and hands on your hips. First go into half camel, reaching back with your right hand to take hold of your right foot. Then come up and reach your left hand to your left foot. Come back up and slowly reach back with both hands to your feet, lifting your chest towards the sky, relaxing your head behind you. Breathe. Come back up by using your abdominal muscles, and sit back onto your heels.

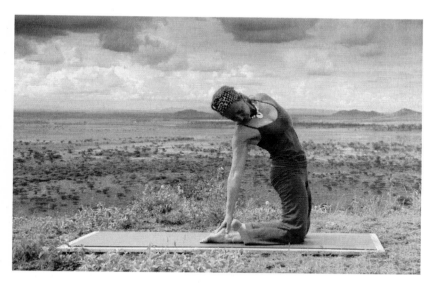

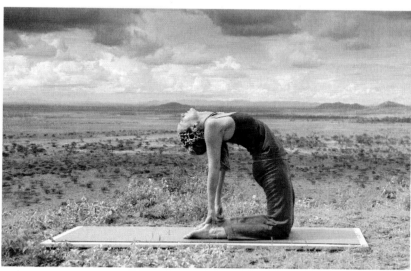

Shoulder Stand and Plow poses.

Lie on your back and bring your knees into your chest. Then touch your feet to the sky, as if you are standing on clouds. You can stay here if you would like, keeping your legs perpendicular to the earth, and your palms down or underneath your hips to support your lower back. If you would like to come into shoulder stand, gently roll up onto your shoulders, supporting your hips with both hands. Keep your upper arms and elbows close to one another on the mat. Your head and neck remain on the mat and your chin is tucked toward your chest with your jaw relaxed. Find your place where you can be comfortable, balanced and relaxed. Most importantly, keep breathing. Then, to move into plow, gently lower your legs behind your head so the tips of your toes are touching the ground, or as far back as you can, using your hands to support the middle of your back. If your toes are touching, clasp your hands together with your arms on the mat. Keep breathing. To come out of these poses, roll out, come to a flat back, relaxing on the ground.

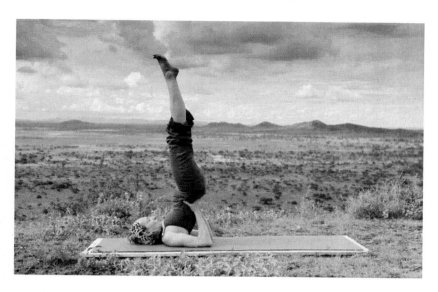

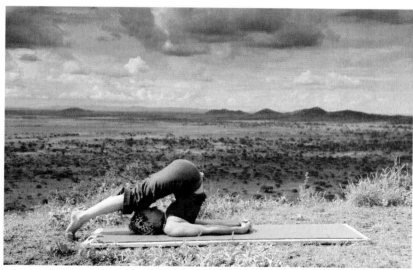

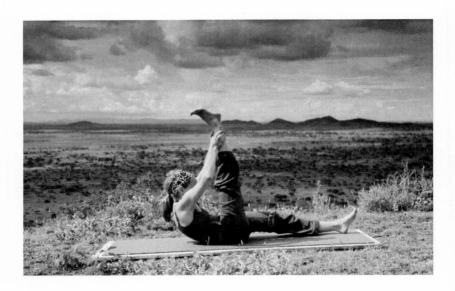

Climb a Tree pose.

From a reclining position, bring your right knee into your chest and then press your right foot towards the sky. Use your hands to climb up your leg, as if you are climbing a tree. Come back down and change legs.

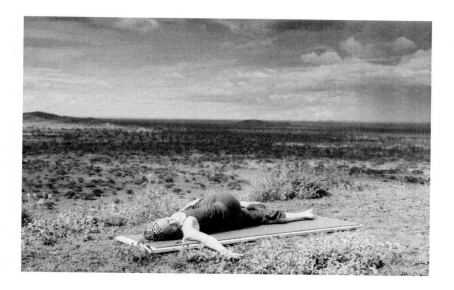

Reclining Twist pose.

From a reclining position, bring your right knee in towards your chest and use your left hand to guide the right knee and leg across your body into a twist. Extend your right arm to the side, keeping your left shoulder on the ground, and look out over your right hand, breath deeply into your lower back. Change sides.

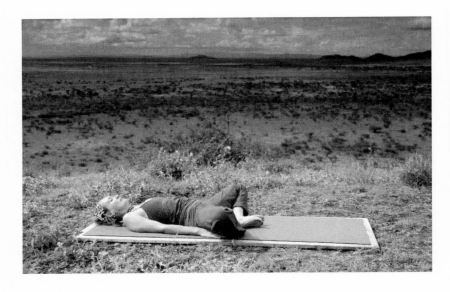

Reclining Butterfly pose.

Lay your body flat upon your mat. Bring the soles of the feet together into a reclining butterfly, breathing into your hips, allowing your knees to relax to your sides. Let your body slowly settle into stillness, allowing the earth to support you. Completely relax into the pose.

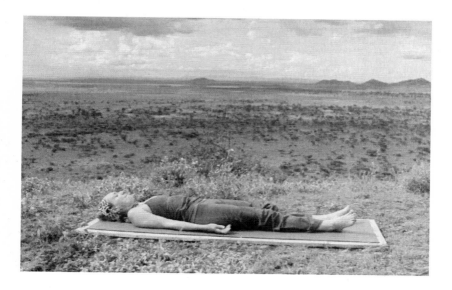

Corpse pose.

Lie on your back with both legs straight, arms along your sides. Close your eyes and let your feet relax. Your palms are facing up towards the sky so you can receive the gifts of the universe. Feel completely supported by the earth. There is no need for effort, just enjoy these moments of stillness.

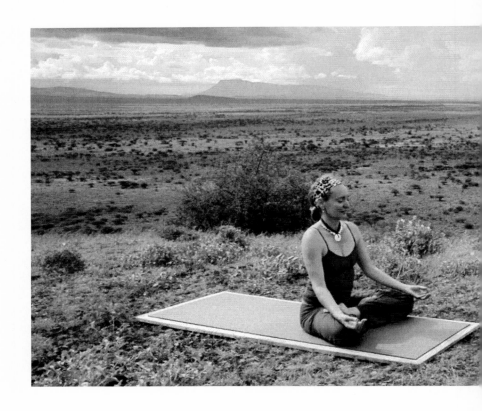

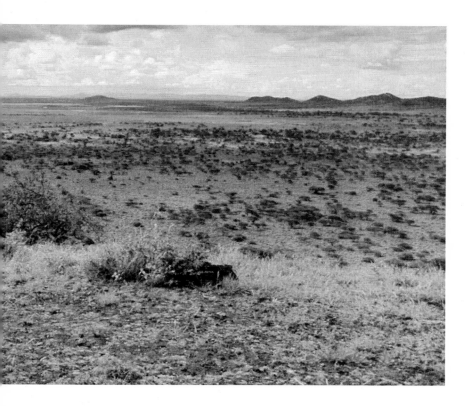

Closing blessing.

It is nice to finish your practice with the same pose you began
with, in this case, a cross-legged position. Close your eyes and feel
how your body feels now, compared to how you began. Take a moment to thank your body for bringing you through this practice.
Honoring the wildlife that we brought into our movements. Bring
your palms together, hands in front of your heart, and say a silent
blessing for all you are grateful for.

7.

Maasai Meditation

The practice of meditation surely originated with the very first people who sat around fires to keep warm. Staring into the flames, in silence, it is easy to slip into other states of consciousness.

Sitting in silence, listening to your nature, has always been a practice in Maasai culture. It is not always easy for those of us living in busy, noisy environments to take the time to sit in silence. Finding a trained meditation teacher will help you learn the right practice and encourage you to keep it. To practice right now, sit comfortably, and close your eyes. Bring your attention inward and become aware of your breath. Repeat the mantra *"ashe,"* meaning 'thank you,' silently to yourself. Whenever you notice that your attention has drifted away from your mantra to other thoughts, sounds, noises, gently bring your attention back to simply repeating *"ashe."*

Sit for fifteen minutes when you begin. You can use a timer with a pleasant chime so that you can relax into your meditation and not worry about missing an activity on your schedule. Gradually add minutes to the time you sit in meditation. To gain the greatest benefits from adding the practice of meditation to your day, find a comfortable place to sit and repeat a mantra with your eyes closed for thirty minutes upon waking in the morning—ideally at sunrise—and again for thirty minutes at sunset. Even if you sit for fifteen to twenty minutes at each session, you will begin to notice changes in your life. Most people find their sleep improves, they feel calmer and they are able to make choices and decisions with greater clarity and confidence. The practice of meditation is timeless; its benefits are profound.

8.

Where Are We?

A MAASAI ELDER SPEAKS,
OLE SULULU IN HIS OWN WORDS

As I mentioned early in this book, the Maasai word *oloipung'o*
means to travel away from your village, explore another part
of the world, then turn back home so you can share what you
learned with your people. It really does. In 2000, I traveled from
the United States to Africa to learn about another part of the
world and have returned home to share with my people. I feel
blessed to have a passion for uncovering the secrets of Maasai
health and happiness, fueled by my desire to learn and share.
And, I feel blessed that the Maasai people welcomed me into
their villages and encouraged me to write down what they were
teaching me. They knew their knowledge was disappearing and
they knew I had the skills to translate it in an understandable
way that would help make a difference in many lives far from
Maasailand. I hope I have succeeded.

On a return trip to Tanzania in October 2011, I spoke with Sululu about his perceptions of the current state of the Maasai people and their culture. Here is the transcript of our conversation, with my questions in italics.

How do you feel personally about the current state of Maasai culture?
Maasai culture is different from other cultures. It depends on what you mean, as we have Maasai in Kenya, Tanzania, Uganda; some live in the bush, some live in town. Many still live their own life and do not like to interact with other tribes. Now the government is trying to interfere, take land, and stop parts of our culture. I would say about forty percent still live the way we used to live, in Ngorongoro area, Karian, Loliondo area, Narok. They still live the original way, and it is a good culture. For example, last week they were unearthing the buried stone, for circumcision for a new age set. I was there, out nearby Lolkisale area. They were very strict about their culture, and I like it, I enjoyed it.

But there are many Maasai who move to town?
Yes, because of the life. Nowadays, others are changing within the culture. I remember twenty years ago Maasai would have to go and steal cows from other tribes. But now they no longer steal, because of the mobile phone, people can call police and catch them. That is one reason they have to come to town, to survive. Try to find a job, like *askaris*, night watchmen, which doesn't pay enough money, because they don't have skills. Maasai are very honest, trustworthy people. I was thinking though, you can't find a Maasai who has been to school who then becomes a watchman.

They learn something else and try to find something else to do after they go to school.

How do you think about your own sons? They don't dress in Maasai clothes, do they?

They don't dress like Maasai because they are already living the history of the town and because of the Christianity. For a long time, they believe that all people who dress like the Western people are Christian, which is not true. That is why we sometimes believe it is the church, or religion, that really destroyed Maasai culture.

I left my home village more than twenty years ago. I am a Maasai, my wife she is a Maasai, but my children were born in town. I have to take them to English-medium schools so they can have a better life. They don't have time to learn the cultural things. It is really painful for me because I believe culture is life. People who don't have a strong culture are like a tree without roots. This is why it is now better to find another way to teach about culture, not in a way that makes children feel like it is a boring old way to live, but it is the nicest life.

If you look at the Kikuyu people in Kenya, many have developed in the modern way but also still are very strict to their culture. Much depends on the government where people live. If a government helps to support the indigenous culture and the people, instead of seeing them as money-making objects, then people will feel good about keeping their traditions.

So you see the impact of Christianity on Maasai culture?

Oh yes. But you know, I think the problem is that many just

don't understand it correctly. For example, in the Bible, if you really read it, Jesus says something like I am not coming to drop the command of God, but I am coming to support you. So people have to live the way they are. Live the natural way, love each other. Try to live with your tribe and try to follow the culture. But people did not get that. They keep using commands, telling people how they should live. It is really a disaster, especially now with all the tribes mixing and following a religious leader. Many people have lost their direction.

So, what do you see as the future of the Maasai?

Well, I can say the Maasai can maybe exist for another ten years in the traditional way. It can be longer if we continue to teach our younger generation about culture, and about taboos. Like how you are supposed to behave and what you are not supposed to do, especially according to your age set. This is really getting lost.

Who does this teaching and how does the teaching happen?

We have the head of a family, the owner of the boma, who traditionally took the time to talk to his sons. That is the first "class." The second class is when you move towards being a warrior, and then elders are chosen to teach. This works in the village, but it is very difficult in town. In town everybody is always running, running, running. Originally a lot of talking happened during the time cows were being grazed or in the evening. We didn't have television. When you were out grazing cows, the young boys would teach each other about medicinal plants, what is used for counteracting snake bites, for example.

Also, in the community we had some people who knew how to read the organs of diseased cows that had died and knew what the cows had died of so we could prevent illnesses from spreading. A lot of this knowledge is gone because we don't live in the traditional way anymore. Somehow these people who go to school to be a veterinarian take a long time to learn these things and often they still don't know enough. We know because we lived it.

I was telling someone in town the other day that I was at a ceremony where they slaughtered two goats, and I asked to see inside the animal whether it looked like it was going to rain this year. You can tell how the goat eats, it prepares for the future. The guy said to me, "You know, Christians are not allowed to do that! You can't look at the meat, we don't believe that." What the elders have taught us is not about beliefs, it is just a sign of the rain. An important sign. This is what I mean about the impact of Christianity sometimes. People misunderstand. Our *Engai* teaches us to use the tools, of the clouds, the wind, the movements of the animals. This is a sign of the past things or the future. This younger generation is not accepting this. It is sad. They are lost.

What other knowledge might be useful for modern people that has more of a chance of being passed on?
Well, for example, the Maasai know how to live together with the wildlife. We work hard to get the food we need and other things from the livestock. Other people in the country kill the wildlife to get money, especially now. The poaching is terrible. We need to educate young people about the importance of wildlife, of keeping the animals alive.

And what about health care?

Well, if you go to remote areas like Serengeti, there are no dispensaries, no Western medicine. Some foreign people donate medicine, but if the Maasais there could really get the support to collaborate with the Western doctors it would be good. The Maasais once knew what medicine was used to cure things. Now many believe a pill is better, which it might be, but still you need to know what is wrong, what really happened, and about side effects.

Any other wisdom from the Maasai with health issues?

Well, we have important traditions according to age and men and women. Normally you see the elder men sitting under an acacia tree talking, or women sitting together making beads, talking. Warriors taking the cows and talking together, exchanging ideas. This talking relieves stress. You know, Western people have a lot of stress. They try to use the mobile phone and the internet to talk with people to relieve stress, but it just seems to make them crazy. People just jump. Nobody prepares anymore for things. Nobody takes the time really necessary to understand what is happening. You know, sometimes I ask people why they come and try to collect all this money for someone in hospital for medicine when they can go and spend time with the person, sit with them, make a meditation?

Anything else the Maasai can teach us modern folks?

The Maasai are very good at resolving problems. I see many Westerners when they have a problem, they react by provoking the other side: couples, parents, and children. We don't do that.

Living together creates problems. When there is a misunderstanding we have to sit down, and talk. People have to know themselves; who are you and what do you want? Who is your godfather or godmother? Ask people. Western people think their own head is enough, but it is not enough. You need advice, people to process with, your best friend. We have a lot to offer about relationships, resolving things before they get worse. Many people in the world have problems; I can see them when they come to travel here. But they don't know how to resolve problems. They think money can resolve the problem, but that often makes it worse! A guy is very lucky if he has a lot of money and knows himself very well and knows what he has to do exactly to resolve his problem.

Why do you think the Maasai people have succeeded for so long in retaining their culture compared to many other tribes?
    Well, many Maasai have left the country to get educated in Canada, the United States, Germany, China, and other places. They adapt to some culture for a while and then bring it back home. Many come back and say, "It is a better life to live in nature."

What can the world do to help keep alive the important elements of Maasai culture?
    We have a lot of volunteers coming to do vaccinations, teaching about sanitation, and they are helping a lot. If they follow the spirit it will work. It is important to bring visitors to Maasai communities. This helps the indigenous people see how important their culture is, see that people come from far away to be together.

9.

A Final Word

Once you begin practicing profoundly simple and meaningful ways of being in the world, it becomes easy to prioritize your life. Your days are rich with family, friends, and purposeful work. You find your decisions come faster, fill you with greater satisfaction, and you end up having all the time in the world. That is, all the cows in the world—whatever cows mean to you.

I know it is bold to claim it is possible to harness the gems of indigenous wisdom—the stuff that has worked well in traditional cultures over many centuries—and marry them with modern ways of thinking and being that work in today's world. Because I have lived this integration of old and new, indigenous and contemporary, I know it is possible, in essence, to uncover the bushman or woman in all of us, that seed of indigenous consciousness that still lies inside us all. My goal in creating this book is to nurture and nourish it. I have good evidence that it can become something great!

What follows are a variety of resources I recommend to readers who are eager to learn more, to visit Maasailand and experience its wonders firsthand, and to help traditional Maasai culture and its wisdom survive far into the future.

Resources to Learn and Experience More

DVD—Maasai Yoga & Meditation with Tanya Pergola, PhD and music by Pops Mohamed. Filmed on location at the base of Mt. Kilimanjaro this 60-minute DVD features a 30-minute all-levels yoga practice, a 15-minute meditation that takes you on a safari in consciousness, and a conversation with Dr. Tanya and Ole Sululu. You can use this program daily to cultivate strength, balance and peace in your body-mind. The DVD is available at **www.tanyapergola.com**.

People-to-People Safaris, www.peopletopeoplesafaris.com, combine a traditional African wildlife safari with truly authentic and respectful cultural and community experiences. Visitor expenditures from these safaris support the projects of Terrawatu, making People-to-People Safaris one of the only philanthropic safari companies in sub-Saharan Africa. Come on a **Healing Safari**—a destination spa meets wildlife safari experience in the stunning landscapes of Tanzania. Your journey begins in consultation with Dr. Tanya Pergola who co-creates the itinerary with Maasai elder Lekoko Ole Sululu to help you resolve issues such as achieving a healthy weight, de-stress, overcoming addiction, detoxification and healing family problems. Upon arrival in Tanzania, Dr. Tanya and Sululu will guide you on a profoundly peaceful journey that includes: relaxing into primordial African nature, yoga and meditation practice in stunning settings, meetings with spiritual healers, wildlife exploration, delicious organic food from local farms, and participation in Maasai community rituals and ceremonies tailored to your issues. A Healing Safari includes follow-up when you return to your home country to assist you in integrating newfound mind-body wisdom into your daily lifestyle.

Terrawatu, **www.terrawatu.org**, is the organization co-founded in 2000 by Dr. Tanya Pergola and Lekoko Ole Sululu to promote sustainable development in Maasai communities. Terrawatu taps time-tested ancient wisdom together with cutting-edge technology to create development projects rooted in community. Since its founding, Terrawatu has built classrooms, tree nurseries, computer labs, integrated medicine clinics and sponsored the education of girls in Tanzania. Its newest initiatives include income generation projects and project management for Corporate Social Responsibility (CSR) programs. Visit **www.terrawatu.org** to learn more and make donations.

Workshops, Yoga & Meditation classes, and handcrafted products from Tanzania, visit **www.tanyapergola.com**. Experience Maasai healing techniques integrated into workshops, yoga programs and meditation training. Dr. Tanya Pergola is a certified Vedic Master with the Chopra Center, founded by Deepak Chopra. She offers in-depth trainings in Primordial Sound Meditation and the Perfect Health Ayurvedic Lifestyle Program, and teaches the Seven Spiritual Laws of Yoga. Visit the shop at **www.tanyapergola.com/shop** to purchase products handcrafted in Tanzania such as the *Chic Maasai Yoga Mat Bag*, made by a women's cooperative, to carry your yoga mat on all of life's safaris.

Herbal Cleanse Kit, http://herbs4orlpul.shopzrii.com
To conduct your own *orlpul* as described in the chapter "Staying Clean and Clear," it is important to include an herbal cleansing program that works well with your own lifestyle, eating habits, and availability of food in your part of the world. The Zrii Purify Cleanse is an Ayurvedic formulation made with similar plants that are traditionally used by the Maasai, all scientifically tested. It is a gentle cleansing program that includes herbal preparations in capsule form, a good tasting fiber mixture, and a vegetarian oil that works like the animal fat the Maasai use to remove impurities from your fat cells, lubricate the channels of the body and facilitate waste removal. When you reach the website **http://herbs4orlpul.shopzrii.com** click on "Shop Now" and select "Purify—The Total Cleanse System."

Shu'mata Camp, www.shumatacamp.com
Ole Sululu leads the popular, in-depth Maasai experience at this luxury camp on the border of Tanzania and Kenya. Shu'mata—meaning 'at the top of everything' in Maa, the language of the Maasai—is also one of the locations for the Healing Safaris, led by Dr. Tanya Pergola and Ole Sululu. This stunning permanent camp

sits on a hill in the midst of Maasailand with an amazing view of Mt. Kilimanjaro. The land is abundant with medicinal plants, and African wildlife walk the savannah together with the Maasai. This is where you want to be to experience profound peace and well-being in following the rhythms of nature.

Acknowledgments

My deepest gratitude goes to the many loving souls that contributed to the birthing of this book. *Time is Cows* has been a very special project, one that has come to life through the support of my amazing family in the United States and in Africa.

I express special thanks:

- to my teachers Howard S. Becker, Wangari Maathai, David Simon, and Deepak Chopra for your profound advice, guidance and encouragement.

- to Ithateng Mokgoro, Patti Spencer, Lucie Bradley, Bradford Zak, and Scholastica Kimaryo for reading the drafts of the manuscript and providing me with your invaluable inputs.

- to my awesome production team Russell Martin for your incredible editing and Hans Teensma for your brilliant cover and interior design. And to Andreas Sigrist for capturing the cover photo, a magical Maasai moment.

- to Yvette Pergola, my absolutely wonderful mom, and my loyal sister Lara Pergola, for your love and support, and for proofreading the manuscript.

- to the fabulous hosts of Gibbs Farm, Hatari Lodge, and Kimemo Cottages for providing such peaceful and inspiring accommodations for me to complete the first draft of the manuscript, and to the coffee shops where I sat and wrote and used your electricity from generator during the times of power cuts in Tanzania—Caffè Classico, Epi d'or Café and The Arusha Hotel.

- to all of the staff and friends of Terrawatu, who have never stopped believing in me and supporting our vision, especially Mrs. Jen Sululu, Angella Marcel, Dorice Henry and Eddy Sululu.

- to my students and patients who have allowed me to help guide you on your path towards abundant health and happiness. You are why I do what I do.

- to my Chopra Center family and amazing fellow certified instructors around the world who are always there to remind me that together, we can continue to bring more and more light into this world.

- to everybody in my village in Miami, who have welcomed me back into the United States with open arms and hearts, especially Lynn Bretsnyder, Steven Anton Rehage, Nancy Morgan Buell, Rachel McCawley, Frances Rhodis, Lorna Owens, Livia Stabile, Liza Gallardo Walton, Tara Calvani, James Schildknecht, Michael Falsetto, Milda Bublys, Tim Gray, Carlos Martinez and the lovely spirits at Dharma Studio.

- to my soul sisters and brothers—April Linton, Kelo Kubu, Elisabetta Grassia, Senait Mekonnen, Marlies Alpers Gabriel, Diane Brunschwig, Meagan Carmody, Kakuta Ole Maimai,

Anna Jonsson, Stephanie Gailing, Stella Ernst, Mmatshilo Motsei, Jessica Erdtsieck, Catherine Lloyd, Anne Sanders, Jim Corey, Gemma Burford, David Scheinman, Catherine Buan, Amy Brangaccio Wolf, Cate Hamilton Drost, Wendy Compernolle, Stacia Soysal, Lucy and George Vrontamitis, Monica Opole, Roslyn Parker, Susan Gustafson, Lisa Chait, Ian Macfarlane, Frank Artress, Zawadi David, Satya, Elena Jensen, Sara Curran, Clive Harvey Fox, Emmanuel Nyaki, Josephine Simon, Dale Jensen, Stephi Hill, Tamalyn Dallal, Ann Vogel, Stacy Morrison, Bernie Hall, Ronda Zelezny-Green, Peter Ray Mwasha, Lisa Peterson, Helen Peeks, Mark Hutchens, Kerri Gladwin, Erica Fischbach, Kate Paulin, Anja Eva Keller, Maya van der Poel, Anna Lappé, and my 'tribe' in Seattle, Orange County, Connecticut, Milan, Cape Town, Johannesburg, Dar es Salaam, Zanzibar, Arusha and Nairobi. I know how long you all have been waiting for this book. Thank you for your endless support and love.

♦ to the children in my life, especially Moon Mokgoro and Boris Sululu, being your Auntie Tanya means the world to me.

♦ and, most importantly, to my brother, best friend and co-creator of this book, Lekoko Ole Sululu, without you *Time is Cows* would never have been born. *Ashe naleng naleng kaka.*

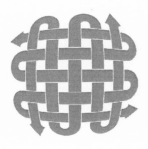

Connect with Dr. Tanya Pergola

Website: **www.tanyapergola.com.**
There is a newsletter sign-up and
Tanya's schedule of workshops, classes and talks.

Email: **tanya@tanyapergola.com**

Facebook: **www.facebook.com/tanya.pergola**

Twitter: **@TanyaPergola**